TWIN STARS AND A MOTHER FROM MARS

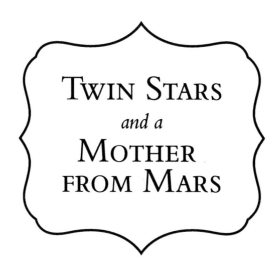

TWIN STARS
and a
MOTHER
FROM MARS

TRU SPENCER

SilverWood

Published in 2013 by the author
using SilverWood Books Empowered Publishing®

SilverWood Books
30 Queen Charlotte Street, Bristol, BS1 4HJ
www.silverwoodbooks.co.uk

ISBN 978-1-78132-126-3 (paperback)
ISBN 978-1-78132-127-0 (ebook)

British Library Cataloguing in Publication Data
A CIP catalogue record for this book is available from the
British Library

Set in Sabon by SilverWood Books
Printed on responsibly sourced paper

For Stanley and Mabel

Contents

Acknowledgements

There are too many people to mention who've helped me in one way or another over the years to achieve my much wanted family. There are, however, a few who are really quite special or whose help and kindness has stayed with me, and will never be forgotten. To those I say a huge thank you:

James, for his never-ending reserves of tolerance, and keeping the faith. My mum and dad for their constant love and support; words will never be enough. Mr Paul Serhal and all the staff at University College Hospital Fertility Clinic, London (now the Centre for Reproductive & Genetic Health) without whose medical expertise we wouldn't have our twin stars – you truly are the best. Anna and Chris Cleland, for their friendship, support and 'meals on wheels'. Daniel Elliott of The London Acupuncture Clinic, Harley Street, London, for being flexible and encouraging. Marie Barnard, midwife, for her genuine concern and reassurance. Oxfordshire Fire & Rescue Service HQ Management Team for their tolerance and understanding. Ali's Pharmacy, London E1, for such a small gesture that meant so much. The labour ward operating theatre team at the John Radcliffe Hospital Oxford, for their efficiency and professionalism. Finally, to Eros Ramazzotti, for making music that touches the soul, which has comforted me through the bad times and celebrated with me during the good, not only during treatment but for the past twenty years.

Introduction

Have you ever thought that maybe you're living on another planet? That's exactly what it felt like when my partner James and I experienced what we consider the most difficult period of both of our lives. We wanted what came easy to so many – a family. I decided to write this book from my diary of events that started in the spring of 2003. It is a completely personal account of the path we took, the gruelling process and sense of isolation that is IVF, and the resulting pregnancy. When I say a personal account I mean that this is from my perspective, not James's, although I'm sure he'd agree with much of what I've written. It is a record of my thoughts, feelings and opinions throughout the whole process and from our experiences with both the NHS and private practice.

This journey has challenged and changed me in many ways – I struggle to describe how and to what depth, but the nearest I can explain is that a part of my soul has disappeared. I'm hardened in my outlook on life. I've felt angry, cheated, hurt – both physically and emotionally, mentally exhausted, upset, lost and probably most of all, lonely. Some of those things I remember to this day amongst other most joyous feelings that made the whole process worth the bad experiences. Maybe my story will help someone trying to make the decision about whether to follow this path. Maybe it will help someone already on it. Maybe the only person it will ever help is me. Whatever your reason for reading my story, I hope you gain an insight and a new respect of the struggle that we, and many others, have been and will continue to go through. I wish you an interesting and thought-provoking read.

Chapter 1

Discovery

Spring 2003

We'd been together since November 1998 – I was thirty-three, James was forty-one. Both of us were working full-time and had good careers. The past few months had seen us evaluate what we really wanted from life and one of those things we both agreed on was that we couldn't imagine not having a family of our own. We'd been saying that it wasn't the right time for what felt like years, and we finally realised that if we kept waiting and waiting and using that as the reason not to then it would never happen. Besides, given that we both wanted more than one child ideally and I was already considered medically 'over the hill', it was now or never if you like, and we decided to start actively trying to make it happen.

I booked us a holiday somewhere warm, making sure the timing was just right. We were both healthy, non-smokers, light drinkers, and we exercised regularly. Couldn't go wrong, we'd be pregnant in no time. At that point I was so excited. Doing the calculations, if I fell pregnant straight away he or she would be a Christmas baby – fantastic!

We flew out to Lanzarote for a week in March. The hotel was amazing – inside the main reception area there was a huge garden with tropical plants and ponds. The grounds were landscaped with mini 'beaches' and canopied sun loungers, and every afternoon at 4 p.m. we were served English tea and biscuits. It was perfect. We just relaxed, read lots of books and concentrated on being together.

On our return home life resumed and we both went to work as normal. I was convinced that I would miss my period so I was very surprised when it arrived on time. I couldn't believe it. How could that have happened? I'd been right in the middle of my cycle and the likelihood of getting pregnant was really high. I was so disappointed and started to wonder what could have gone wrong. Was it me? Was it James? Were we just unlucky? Although I knew that it took on average several months to conceive, I had just naïvely assumed we'd hit the jackpot first time. My mind started whirring and doubts set in – thinking about it, we'd been together so long and nothing had ever happened in spite of me not taking the Pill and not using protection, but somehow I suppose I just didn't imagine there'd be a problem. I thought it must be me and that there was something wrong. I was too old, I worried too much and I needed to relax more. All sorts of reasons entered my head, but I decided that I was being silly and that really it would just take a bit of time, especially given our ages. James didn't even question why I wasn't pregnant straight away; he was much more philosophical about it all. We decided that we'd just get on with things and give it until early the following year before we started worrying about something that was probably not relevant anyway.

Sometime during September I came across a book called *Taking Charge of Your Fertility* by Toni Weschler[i]. I thought it would be worth a go so read it cover to cover and afterwards felt completely energised and positive and that it was the answer to our problem. I thought I'd wait until after Christmas, given that we said we'd just let nature take its course and not interfere until the following year. However, January 2004 arrived and still nothing, so I started to keep note of my morning temperatures by using the charts supplied in the back of the book – just before an egg is released body temperature increases ever so slightly, and if it could be detected it enabled you to pinpoint the most fertile days.

On the chart I had to fill in the first day of my period with the date and day of the week and take my temperature on waking, before even getting out of bed, meaning I had to keep a thermometer on the bedside table. I also monitored cervical fluid to see whether it was sticky, creamy, or like 'egg-white', as this also changes according to fertility. As well as this I logged any exercise taken, any illness, stress, drugs taken (such as paracetamol for instance), travel and any other comments that I thought might be relevant. Little did I know then but it was just the start of what would become a completely mechanical process, when the focus was always on timing and a tense two week wait to see if my period would put in an appearance. Which it always did of course; every single month. Each time I would try and stay positive thinking this time it was right, this time I was pregnant. Then the inevitable disappointment came when I had the signs that meant I knew I'd get my period. I started to worry and 'what ifs' entered my head. What if things were so bad that we couldn't have a family at all, ever? What if we had to do some sort of IVF treatment? I'd often thought about it but didn't honestly think it would apply to me. It suddenly started to dawn on me that it could be a reality.

Somehow though I managed to convince myself that everything would be OK and it was still just an issue of timing. I carried on with the charting, trying to get on with life in the meantime, in the hope that if I didn't think about it too much then it would work. Of course, it was impossible for me to not think about it. It was always in my thoughts – I'd never been very good with letting things occur and just waiting to see. I prefer to at least have a rough idea of what's going to happen and when. Dealing with all this uncertainty felt very strange to me and I found it difficult to comprehend.

It was quite a struggle to focus, but as the days went by we did all the usual things we liked to do – getting up mid-morning on a Saturday, going into Oxford to read the papers and magazines whilst having a coffee and lunch, spending a couple of hours relaxing – James in his 'shed' (a bookshop), me wandering the shops just browsing, then returning home for dinner and either a DVD, or maybe the cinema. We didn't have a huge social circle. We'd both moved around too much to stay in touch with a large group of friends and, after working hard all week, we just wanted to relax doing our own thing.

It was during one of these lazy weekends in early spring that I heard a radio advertisement for local couples wanting to become pregnant in the near future to take part in a free trial at the local hospital. Initially it didn't register that this could be something that might help us so I didn't really pay much attention to it. I heard it several times throughout the following week and thought that next time it came on the radio I'd jot down the number. Over the next few days I kept listening but to my frustration I never heard the advert again. I wondered how I could find out the information – I tried calling the radio station but no joy there. I finally thought it may be worth contacting the hospital directly so I called in, explained what I'd heard, and was immediately put through to the public health department. They knew exactly what I meant as they were running the trial so I was asked to go in and see them. It all happened quickly – I went in a couple of days later and, after being assessed for health and background checks, emerged with something that I thought would solve everything.

What I'd been given was a fertility monitor. It worked in much the same way as the manual temperature taking method that I'd been used to, except it was an ovulatory hormone that was being measured. Every morning I had to pee on a stick similar to those in pregnancy test kits, then insert it into the monitor for a few moments where it registered the hormone level for the day. It then told you when you were about to ovulate and were most likely to become pregnant. That would be several days every month, and once you saw the egg symbol on the monitor it was your sign to get active! It was a lot easier than temperature taking, although I still did that too, just as a double check. I think at that point James thought things were getting a bit too mechanical, although he was happy for me to carry on using the monitor. It wasn't doing any harm and it wasn't a drug that I was taking so in terms of my health there were no issues. To be honest, it took some of the stress out of things – I wasn't relying totally on myself as the machine took all the responsibility for logging what was happening, so I actually managed to relax more.

The trial was being run for a total of six months, during which time the majority of women were expected to become pregnant. I started it in April 2004. By September 2004, guess what? Still no pregnancy, so I made an appointment to see the nurse at the hospital. She printed out a chart for me from the information stored on the unit (I'd had to insert a special card at the end of every month that recorded each month's findings). It told me that my cycle was fairly regular, if a bit lengthy, and I was ovulating normally every month. I was given the option of continuing by using another unit via a sister trial that was being run by the manufacturers of the system. Of course I jumped at the chance, still thinking at that point that we were just being unlucky. It was amazing how much I convinced myself that luck was the only thing that played a part in something that should've been blindingly obvious. It seemed that I didn't really want to accept that things weren't as they should be. I hoped that it would just be a bit longer, and we'd be pregnant, although I think I knew really that we'd come to the end of the road of anything happening naturally and that we needed medical investigations. I thought, OK, I'm still young enough, no problem. Let's do another six months with this new unit, then if nothing happens we'll take the next step.

October, November, December 2004. Three months on and no result. I couldn't carry on with this for another three months – quite clearly it wasn't going to happen. It was time to have a conversation about what to do next. When I say that, I think what I really meant was 'we need to go to the doctor for investigations and I'm making the appointment'. I think James really knew that was what we needed to do but from a male perspective, taking that step probably felt like admitting to failure and I'm sure it was quite difficult for him, as it could reveal outcomes that neither one of us would want to face. We did agree, however, to wait until after Christmas, so I made an appointment for the following January 2005 with our GP.

Christmas came and went. We did the usual – travelled up to James's parents' house for Christmas Eve, then over to my parents' late Christmas Day for a couple of days. Nothing out of the ordinary – just some quiet family time. I always took a couple of weeks off at this time of year to just relax, read books and sleep! We didn't usually plan on doing anything for New Year's Eve – all too over-hyped. Maybe it was an age thing – we'd had our fair share of partying and clubbing over the years, but that gave way to serious work and pure relaxation a couple of years ago. I tried not to think about things too much for a few weeks. Having made an appointment I felt that we were finally doing something in the right direction.

January 2005

It was mid month and we were due to see the GP. He went through our histories, asked us how long we'd been actively trying, and whether I had regular periods. James was examined and the doctor said he could find nothing physically wrong, so the next step was a sperm analysis and count. James was given a small pot and instructions about getting it to the hospital on the morning he provided the sample, still kept warm, so it could be analysed. We left the GP's office slightly bewildered. James looked a bit odd. I had no idea what was going through his head at that point; probably that it was all a bit of a waste of time, but he did agree to carry on as he knew how important it was to me. Hopefully it was important to him too, but you didn't often know with James – he wasn't always very good at showing how he really felt.

A couple of days later I dropped the pot off at the hospital. It felt rather strange taking the lift up to one of the top floors and walking down the corridor with a sample pot in my pocket. I also found it a bit awkward handing it in to the woman behind the small hatch in the laboratory. I don't know why, although it felt like there was a stigma attached, and it all felt so private. The lab assistants would know why I was there – I thought they'd laugh or give knowing looks. It didn't really register in my mind that to them it was part of a normal day and they'd done this a thousand times before. I think at that point I realised that this would be the start of well-meaning prying of strangers into something that should really be so personal. Being an introverted and private person, I found the thought of that rather alarming.

We'd been told that it would take a week or so before the results of the test would be available, and around eight days later we received a letter asking us to phone the GP's surgery. I knew that they didn't send results such as this in the post, so it didn't seem odd at all. I thought that if there was a problem it would be with me, trying to ignore the small niggling voice in my head that was telling me this wouldn't be the case.

It was late in the afternoon when I finally managed to contact the GP. Our usual doctor was away that day, so the receptionist asked me if I wanted to speak to someone else. Well, of course, I wanted confirmation that everything was OK and normal, so I spoke to one of the female doctors instead. She came on the phone quite cheerful and proceeded to tell me that the results had come back. She said that the sample count had been a bit low, and the quality was a bit worse than they would normally expect. However, she said that often the sample wasn't taken to the hospital in time, or it got too cold in transit, both of which would be detrimental. She told me not to worry, and that if I went by the surgery to pick up another pot we could send in another sample as a comparison test.

I felt a bit sick and started to panic. I tried to run through it all again, tried to think about it with my head, not my heart, but I was unable to be objective. I agreed to go and pick up another pot. We'd do another sample. I called James and told him. He was a bit taken aback and it went very quiet on the other end of the phone. I think he probably also started to worry. He said that he couldn't see any reason why there should be a problem. He'd never smoked, didn't drink much, was healthy...I said that if there was a problem it was more than likely something he couldn't do anything about. I tried to convince him that the second sample would be fine, then we'd move on to investigating me more.

However, I really didn't think it was me. I already knew at this point that the second sample would reveal the same thing. And I was right. Actually, the second time around it was worse. The count had decreased and the quality wasn't great either. There was our answer. After all this time we had our reason. It was quite a shock when faced with the reality and I wasn't sure what to do next. I managed to speak to our usual GP who was very pragmatic about it. He made an appointment for me to get some bloods done to check my hormone levels etc. and for me to see a fertility consultant to review whether there was also a problem with me. As with many things concerning the NHS, this was going to take time. I decided that this was something we didn't have, given our ages, so I paid to see the same consultant privately within a week.

I saw him at the private Manor Hospital, next door to the NHS one in Oxford. What a difference. Waiting for the consultant, it felt like I was in a smart hotel; quiet atmosphere, carpeted floors, drinks on tap (well, beverages anyway). I even managed to park my car in the underground car park for free.

My appointment was an evening one, and unfortunately the consultant was running late – some things didn't change, regardless of whether you went private or not. I remember sitting in the waiting room thinking how appalling it was that I'd paid over £100 and they still couldn't run the show on time. Never mind. I perused the magazines and watched the clock.

I was finally called in at around 7 p.m. The consultant was very pleasant. He quickly reviewed the results of the sperm analyses. My blood results had also arrived and didn't reveal anything out of the ordinary. Again, he was quite matter of fact about it. That was his job I suppose, seeing lots of people with infertility problems. He was just very business-like – not particularly warm or friendly, but not cold or rude either. He asked if I had any other questions, which at that point I didn't, apart from what the next step would be. He confirmed that if we wanted to pursue having a biological family, we would need fertility treatment.

It would be the type recommended for male factor infertility called ICSI – intracytoplasmic sperm injection, a technique in which a single sperm is injected into an egg to fertilise it.

He said that he would refer us to the Oxford Fertility Unit at the John Radcliffe Hospital. We could expect a letter which would give us the next available dates of an infertility open evening that we would need to attend before deciding whether to go ahead. As he was talking I managed to be quite professional and 'in the moment'. I didn't really react to what he said. I just sat there nodding and saying, yes, yes, OK. No problem. Thank you very much.

The appointment over, I left the room and walked back to my car, deep in thought. It was about 8 p.m. I was on my own in a quiet, deserted hospital and I'd just been told that we'd need fertility treatment to have a family. I felt numb. I reflected back over my life and realised that I always felt that it wouldn't be straightforward when it came to having a family. I can't explain why. I just always knew that was how it would be. Some may say that was just negative thought because I'd been put in just that situation. I don't think so though. My gut feeling had been pretty accurate about most things to date.

I arrived back home on what must have been auto-drive to tell James. When I told him I tried to stay rational but couldn't manage it. I just cried. I cried from the stress of the past few years, I cried because I felt awful for him being told the news that it was male factor infertility, I cried because I felt sorry for myself. And I cried because I knew that we were at the beginning of a hard road. The past few years of trying for a family would be nothing compared to what was in store.

Chapter 2

Expectation

February 2005

So we had our diagnosis. The thought of IVF treatment was constantly in my mind and it was difficult to concentrate on anything else. I found myself getting carried away with what the future might hold. Somehow I had to get a grip on my feelings and try to be more detached and practical. But how could I detach myself from the thought that maybe I wasn't going to have a family? Ever. Potentially never carry a baby, give birth, hold and comfort my child, watch him or her grow? It was almost too unbearable to think about. All I could do was try and take it one step at a time and deal with each outcome as and when it happened. I tried to throw myself into my studies that I was doing in my free time. Sometimes it worked. Sometimes I just wanted to do nothing. It felt a bit like wallowing and the guilt set in. Maybe it would all work out anyway so what was the point of being negative and depressed about it at this early stage? Statistically we had a great chance and it was with this in mind that I prepared myself for the coming days, weeks, and months.

However, I was conscious that there was still something we had to do. Something that I was not looking forward to at all – telling the parents. Up to that point we'd done everything completely alone and had told no-one. I didn't like many people knowing such private information, so dealing with the situation so far had been done 'in-house' so to speak. I decided to drive the several hours to visit my parents for the weekend, hoping I'd get the opportunity to say something. At that point James didn't want to tell his parents so I left it entirely up to him when he chose to do so. The only thing I did insist on was that he should let them know soon or I would find it quite difficult having to put on a 'happy face' each time we saw them to prevent them from asking if there was anything wrong. He agreed, and I knew he'd tell them before any treatment actually started.

I can remember being in my mum's kitchen when I got the chance to speak to her alone. My dad had gone off in the garden somewhere and there'd already been a couple of opportunities to say something but I hadn't plucked up the courage. I don't know what I was so worried about. I suppose I felt a bit like a failure. My life had been quite eventful already, and I think my mum despaired of me sometimes. I didn't know how she would take it, or whether she'd be able to deal with it. Quite why I was worried about that I don't know. All I needed to be concerned about was how I was going to deal with it, not other people. Still, it was important to me that we had my parents' support – it was difficult enough as it was and I think I needed someone else to know to ease my mind a little. I had to tell them at some point, and that needed to be sooner rather than later.

We were sat at the kitchen table having coffee and I just said that I had to tell her something. I kept the tone of my voice quite low, or she'd have thought that I was actually pregnant! Anyway, I just said that we wanted to start a family and unfortunately we had to have fertility treatment. She gave me a hug and started to get upset for me. I explained the reasons why, then we talked about what had happened so far, that we'd been through the investigations already, and how it was definitely what we needed to do to have a family. She was very pensive and I felt as though I'd let her down. So far there were no 'blood' grandchildren; I knew she wanted it so much and there I was telling her that it possibly might never happen.

I asked her to tell my dad for me – I didn't want to go through the act of saying it all over again; it was already emotionally draining. She said she didn't mind and I think she told him when I was in the shower. I could see he was worried but he didn't really mention it to me directly. He was probably at a loss for words.

I found it quite a relief once I'd told them as it meant that I no longer had to deal with it by myself – James aside of course. However, we both decided that we didn't want anyone else to know, other than our parents and our friends Anna and Chris. It was too personal to us, and whilst some people gain comfort from telling everyone what they're going through, I would have just found that too intrusive.

It was at this time that my mum also told me about my cousin and his wife. They'd been trying for a family for several years too, and had recently been offered a free IVF cycle through their local hospital. It was great that they didn't have to worry about the cost but for us, unfortunately, that wasn't necessarily an option – ours could be around £3,000. If it turned out that we had to pay it would annoy me immensely; it would be so inequitable given we'd paid into the system like everyone else. I knew though that there'd be nothing we could do about it and that was that. We were very lucky – my mum had some savings she insisted that we use if we needed to, which was a fantastic thing to do, and I would never be able to thank her enough.

March 2005

We finally received the information about the open evening, scheduled for 5 p.m. one Wednesday in April. We also received a letter from the fertility unit in Oxford that told us about some routine blood tests we had to have before any treatment could start, and which drugs I would have to take. I thought it was a little strange given that we hadn't even been to the open evening yet, but after calling one of the nurses I was told that it was quite normal to start doing all the background checks to save time, as it was a long enough process to begin with.

When I reviewed the letter in more detail I saw that the tests we had to have were numerous – for me they were: full blood count; liver function test; renal profile; serum progesterone; plasma prolactin; plasma testosterone; plasma TSH level; plasma sodium; plasma potassium; plasma creatinine; plasma ALT; plasma albumin; plasma bilirubin; plasma alkaline phosphatase; erythrocyte sedimentation rate; plasma glucose level; HBs antigen; HepC antibody; and HIV antibody. All that and we hadn't even started treatment! As for James he had the last three in the same list plus sperm count and motility. The sight of James's horrified face when they took the blood would be forever etched in my mind; he looked like a ghost and I honestly thought he was going to faint. He'd only had a single vial taken too – I must've had about five! Still, it was compulsory and had to be done before we could proceed. The results all came back with no problems, with the exception of the sperm count. All we had to do was wait for the open evening meeting, and then hopefully we could get going with the treatment cycle.

April 2005

I can remember the drive to the hospital for the open evening, not that it was eventful but because we both sat in complete silence the whole way, lost in our own thoughts. I would get to know the route so well – through Headington, right at the traffic lights, down the hill to the mini roundabout then the third exit into the grounds of the John Radcliffe. This time, though, we went to the private hospital situated next door – the same one I went to for my consultation several weeks earlier, so we didn't have to worry about finding a space in the overcrowded main hospital car park.

We parked the car and entered the lobby area where we were handed an A4 envelope containing a bundle of information relating to the process. I looked around the room and was surprised to see tea, coffee and biscuits on offer. It felt like a group therapy session, which in a way I suppose it probably was. We chose our refreshments then sat down and studied the contents of the envelope which contained details about the types of procedures and the different drugs, although it was all very generic as it wasn't yet tailored to individual requirements. As I skimmed through the information pack I noticed that a lot of couples had arrived in the meantime. Who'd have thought it would be so popular?! Sometimes all you can do is joke about things. In general, fertility treatment is seen as something of a luxury and not a core requirement of provision on the NHS. As it's not life-threatening, like cancer for instance, people often tend to see it as a lifestyle choice, rather than a distressing medical problem. It's a huge drain both on the emotions and the physical body and I found that joking about it sometimes helped to take the pressure off.

We were all herded into a large room with a projector, where someone proceeded to tell us all about the fertility unit, who was who etc., then showed us a film about the process and what was involved. Afterwards we were given the chance to ask questions. Not that I asked any. James didn't either, although several people did. A couple of questions still come to mind, which were something like "How do you know you're fertilising the right egg with the right sperm?" and "How often does it go wrong?"

They were probably prompted by recent media articles that said a couple had an embryo put back that wasn't theirs. The doctor's answer was quite straightforward – they would ask for name, address and date of birth before every single appointment, ensuring that everything matched up with their files and laboratory samples. A tedious but necessary part of the process to make sure everyone knew the couple being treated were who they were supposed to be. For some reason I wasn't worried about that at all. It didn't even enter my head – I believed we just had to trust in the experts to do their job correctly.

Another question was about cost – we were all told that there was no more funding available for treatment on the NHS. Aah, I thought, now we're getting down to it. Not that cost would be a barrier for us – we'd fund it somehow or other, probably with the money my mum had offered. The thing that annoyed me the most was the NHS lottery system, where people in different parts of the country got funding and others didn't. In our area the hospital's budget had been depleted, so it was tough luck. The unit was, however, part-funded, which meant that I could get the medications through the hospital pharmacy, and only pay directly for the actual treatment. At least it was something, and better than having to pay privately for the cost of the drugs. Besides, maybe we'd be lucky and get pregnant from the first round of treatment.

At the group meeting we also received the details of James's assessment appointment and our pre-treatment consultation: Thursday 12th April, followed by the consultation on Tuesday 17th April. It cost £165 for James's analysis appointment, and £120 for the new patient consultation. Both appointments were at the fertility unit at the John Radcliffe Hospital – an environment we would get to know quite well. We had to take some time off work so that we could attend the appointments as there was no choice of day or time; you just had to fall in with whatever you were given, or you had to rearrange for an alternative to be allocated. Luckily we were in a position where we could arrange our working lives around appointments so this element didn't really affect us, although it would have been very difficult for most people in nine-to-five jobs.

Going home that night I felt a real sense of hope and

expectation – a feeling that I'd experience many times throughout the process, along with the inevitable 'crash' and pain of events that would not turn out as we thought. Little did I know at that point what was in store. Those first feelings of hope lifted my spirits and my naïve positivity allowed my head to start rushing ahead of things and begin planning everything 'baby'. If I knew then what I did many, many months later, I would have put the brakes on getting carried away – what is it they say about hindsight?

May 2005

I'd started a new job recently – part-time, no stress, lovely people. I worked from 8.15 a.m. until 1 p.m. as a personal assistant for the fire service. It was something that I had plenty of experience of and it was just the thing I needed whilst going through treatment. I hadn't planned it that way – I'd previously been working full-time for a different company, and as a self-employed administrator on a part-time basis. Several months had passed since I'd resigned from my full-time position – not because of treatment, as I didn't know at that point, but for other personal reasons – travelling so far every day being one of them. It was just the right time to leave. Sometimes I really do think things happen in a particular order that can't be controlled or arranged, and I believed that this was one of those circumstances.

Shortly after the group meeting the hospital called us to arrange for something called a saline scan – sterile saline solution is injected into the cavity of the uterus which then distends, or enlarges it, allowing for accurate measurements to be taken and for the identification of any

31

abnormalities. I decided that it wasn't necessary for James to be there this time; I was quite happy to do it on my own. We'd be discussing all the nitty-gritty of what was involved from a female biology perspective, so he'd probably have felt out of place anyway.

It wasn't a very uncomfortable procedure to go through, quite similar to having a smear test really, and everything looked normal which meant that we could proceed with treatment. I left the hospital in a good mood and after making my way back to my car I decided to go to the gym for an hour or so. I tried to go at least three times a week – it allowed me to have some thinking time without other distractions. Of course I always ended up thinking about the treatment and what it involved and I wondered whether it was still alright to exercise so intensely whilst going through the procedure. Would I be too tired? Would it affect egg production? Would I be overdoing it? All were questions I really hadn't thought about previously. I kept going over it in my head – maybe exercising was good and increased blood flow which would be no bad thing, but then again, maybe it would be too much and I'd be diverting my energy when it was needed elsewhere?

Such little things suddenly started to become big things; started to be the 'thing' that would mean the treatment would work or not. It was completely irrational, and I kept trying to remind myself that I was thinking way too deeply about it all, but I just couldn't help it. I convinced myself in the end that easing up on the exercise wouldn't be detrimental, but it could be if I carried on as intensely as usual. I decided to decrease the effort of each session down to a very slow jog, a leisurely cross-training session, and very light weight training. More than anything, even if it would've been OK to carry on as before, I was more comfortable with taking it easy, and as that meant less worrying it was worth it.

About a week after my saline scan I was at work when a colleague telephoned in to say she had mumps. Apparently someone else had also been off for a couple of days with the same symptoms. Oh dear. My mind started working overtime, again. I was really concerned that I might catch mumps as well; I couldn't remember whether I'd had them as a child, so didn't know if I was immune or not. I tried to think logically – I hadn't been in contact with either of those concerned recently, and as they were off ill the likelihood that I would contract anything was quite small. However, there was still a niggle in the back of my mind so in the end I decided to call the hospital to ask their opinion. I spoke to one of the nurses and told her that I couldn't remember whether I'd already had it, so we had a chat about the possibilities and whether the treatment cycle would be affected if I did get it. All I could do was monitor any potential symptoms and call back if I noticed anything unusual. We still had quite a few weeks before I was due to start with the drugs anyway, so if anything was going to happen we would know before then. I tried not to worry about it and attempted to focus on work and my studies.

Thursday, 12th May 2005
James had a hospital appointment today so his sample could be tested again, confirming the original results. It was a more accurate test as there'd be no time delay before

it could be analysed, given that we didn't have to transport it to the hospital. We met in Oxford afterwards and went to our usual haunt – Starbucks @ Borders. We practically lived there in our spare time, reading the magazines whilst having a coffee.

It was then that James said he was going to tell his parents when they came down to see us at the weekend. I think he was a little nervous at telling them though, naturally enough. We were in Marks and Spencer's coffee shop when he casually mentioned it whilst I was at the counter ordering the drinks. There was a strange silence at the table when I sat down, then his mum mentioned that James had just told them we needed treatment. She seemed quite confused by the whole thing, so I started to explain why and what had happened so far. She couldn't understand why there would be a problem and said that James had always eaten well, never smoked or had any other health issues, so why should he have a problem in this department? I tried to explain as best I could, but it was quite hard to get her to understand that if we wanted a biological family we had no choice. I told them both that there was no guarantee the treatment would work, and that we just had to go through it and hope for the best outcome. Still not grasping the notion of needing help to have children, they asked me why it shouldn't work. I tried to explain the science behind the treatment and that whilst it increased our chances it wasn't a given. In the end I think they just accepted it. We didn't really speak about it a great deal after that point. For sure, there was the occasion when they'd ask James how things were going, and if I picked up the phone when either of them called they asked if everything was OK. I think it was quite a difficult concept for them to grasp, and they probably just didn't know what to say.

Tuesday, 17th May 2005

A couple of days after James told his parents we were due back at the fertility unit for our consultation with the specialist. Located on the 4th floor of the Women's Centre, it was accessed by a side entrance to the main hospital – ironically the same one that all the pregnant women used for their antenatal appointments. Faced with pregnant women standing outside the entrance smoking cigarettes made my blood boil. I didn't take it personally, but it did make me really angry every single time I saw it, regardless of how often that was.

Once inside the hospital we made our way to the 4th floor via the lift, along with doctors, nurses and patients. On future occasions it would be new parents with their babies in cots, or pregnant women in labour walking round in their slippers. No room for potential hurt feelings here. This element of the process had probably not even been considered. To someone not going through IVF, it wouldn't even occur to them. At the end of the day we were being treated in a general hospital, as most NHS provision for IVF is, and the emotional impact of that was completely unavoidable.

We registered our names with the lady on the reception desk and sat down to wait. The staff had tried to make the area as welcoming as possible – there were magazines, a water fountain, a drinks machine and potted plants, and there was always a radio playing – BBC Radio 2, I think.

There was also a miniature desk and chairs and some toys – it's funny but it's often default thinking that there's an assumption that everyone being treated is childless, when in actual fact that's not always the case. Secondary infertility, when couples find that suddenly they can't get pregnant again, is quite a common occurrence. However, today there were just couples; quite a lot of them actually. It was obviously a very busy department.

I sat quietly and tried to read my book – every time a doctor or nurse came out of a room with a clipboard I thought it was our turn and looked up expectantly, only to hear another couple's names called out. We ended up sitting there for about half an hour until finally we were called and led into a small side room next to the waiting area. It was a tiny space and contained a couple of chairs, a desk, and a computer. Someone who we thought was a nurse asked us to confirm our names and address, then proceeded to tell us that before we went in to see the consultant we had to give her a cheque for £120. I was slightly taken aback as it was completely unexpected. What I mean by that is that whilst we knew we had to pay, the way in which we were herded into a separate room before being allowed to see anyone was rather odd. It appeared calculated somehow, and very impersonal.

Once we'd handed over the money and after our details had been updated onto the computer and we were given a receipt, we were asked to sit back down in reception until the doctor came for us. We'd been waiting ages already, so I supposed another half an hour wouldn't matter.

We both sat down resignedly and I started to leaf through a magazine. A minute or so later, the consultant appeared and showed us through to a different room just off the main corridor. He introduced himself as Mr Child and welcomed us to the unit. He said that he'd read our notes from my first appointment with the consultant, then began to explain the results of James's tests. It all confirmed that we did indeed need to have a type of IVF called ICSI. It was nothing that we didn't know beforehand so, so far, no surprises.

Or at least there weren't, until we were told about two more tests that James had to have – karyotyping and cystic fibrosis screening. The point of these tests was to check if the reason for the low count was genetic; if it was it could help us to decide whether the level of risk to any future children would be acceptable or not. This came as a bit of shock, as up until this point no-one had even mentioned these extra tests before. It wasn't a problem in itself, it was just that we were told we wouldn't be able to start any treatment until after the results came back, and that took approximately two months! It meant even more waiting when we really thought we'd be able to just get on with things. It was disappointing and I was upset. We asked why we hadn't been advised before, and why the procedure for these tests hadn't already been done to prevent further waiting at a time when we'd been led to believe we could start the programme straight away. Of course, there was no answer to this and I got the impression that no-one had really questioned it before, and that most people just accepted it. I started to get the first inkling of what may be in store, and how 'not' in control we were going to be.

The appointment ended and James went off to get more blood drawn. We handed over another £200 for the screening then headed home in silence, going over everything again in our heads. We could do nothing more until the test results came back.

A few days after the consultation, and still irritated by the apparent lack of expediency, I gave the unit a call to discuss how disappointed we were about having to wait so long for the results, and whether it was possible to pay extra to get the tests done privately. I was told there wasn't a lot they could do, although a nurse did offer to contact the company doing the tests to see if they could turn them round any quicker. They couldn't promise, but they said they'd try and push ours to the front of the queue, so hopefully it would only take four or five weeks, instead of seven or eight. With nothing more we could do to influence the process, we just left it in their hands, hoping that it wouldn't be long before we had some news.

Tuesday, 14th June 2005
We received a call from the unit – the blood tests had come back showing no abnormalities. At last we could officially start treatment.

Chapter 3

The Beginning

Late June 2005

On the first day of my period I phoned the unit as the administration of the drugs had to be timed from that point onwards.

Between the 14th and 17th day I went back to the hospital where I was given a more detailed schedule, and a nurse showed me how to do the injections by demonstrating the procedure on an orange! I also collected my drugs from the pharmacy and made the full payment for the treatment – £3,273.

Wednesday, 13th July 2005

Twenty-one days after my period started I began to take the first drug. It was called Synarel and was in the form of a nasal spray, similar to those you use when you have a cold. The aim was to temporarily shut down my ovaries so that my cycle could be controlled by blocking the link with the pituitary gland in the brain, preventing premature ovulation.

This part of the treatment was called 'down-regulation' and it was incredibly important to time the sniffing of the spray very accurately, as to miss or significantly delay it could also delay the next stage of treatment. Timing was everything. I had to do one sniff in each nostril twice per day, so I decided to go with 7 a.m. and 7 p.m. The first time I was incredibly nervous, although I'm not sure why, I could hardly get it wrong. I just looked at the box for a few moments as thoughts went through my mind about taking such heavy-duty drugs. The information sheet inside said there could be strong side effects including headache, rash, acne, hot flushes, myalgia, decrease in bone density, ovarian cysts, itching, vaginal dryness, shortness of breath, chest pain, changes in sex drive, and reduction in breast size – just a few things to think about then! I found it quite difficult to voluntarily introduce something like that into my body when I'd always avoided the usual types of toxins such as smoking, drinking and eating the wrong things. For goodness sake, I only ever took a paracetamol if I really had to, so I struggled to accept that I had to do something that could be so detrimental to my health. Common sense prevailed though – it was only temporary, and there would be no lasting effects. It just had to be done.

I tipped the bottle back and took both sniffs straight after each other. I immediately felt a horrid tasting liquid trickling down the back of my throat. It was an awful, chemical taste and I had to drink some orange juice straight afterwards to take away the foul residue in my throat. Evidently I needed to toughen up – if I found this part difficult I'd be a complete mess by the end.

And so it was, every day for the next few weeks. At some point during the down regulation process I was told to expect a bleed, similar to a period – a withdrawal bleed caused by my hormones reaching a base level. Although it could happen at any time after starting the drugs it usually put in an appearance around the time a normal period would've been expected. It was often heavier than normal though, and could sometimes last longer. Once this had happened and I'd had a blood test confirmed as baseline, the injection of stimulation drugs could begin.

Monday, 1st August 2005
I continued to use the nasal spray for about three weeks, and had the bleed as predicted. I made my way to the hospital for a 2 p.m. blood test appointment to check my hormone levels. It took about ten minutes from arriving to leaving, then I had to wait until the next day to know whether I could start injecting the stimulation drugs.

As promised, I received a telephone call the following morning confirming that I could proceed and advising me that I should start injecting 150iu of 'GonalF' (gonadatrophin) starting on what was referred to as day one, Thursday, 4th August 2005. These drugs stimulated the ovaries to produce eggs so that there'd be enough to 'harvest' at egg collection. During the injections, done at the same time each day, I also had to keep sniffing the down-regulation drug, so the eggs wouldn't be released too soon. After a week of injections I'd have a blood test and ultrasound scan to check for hormone levels and to see how many follicles were maturing. As soon as several follicles had reached 20mm in diameter then a date for egg collection could be arranged.

Faced with having to, I began to wonder whether I'd be able to actually stick a needle in my own skin. I'd read all about how it could really hurt and what to do to dull the pain on many internet sites about infertility. Too much information, definitely. I just had to do it without thinking. One thing less to worry about in this respect was that the drugs were administered by way of a special 'pen'. The liquid was already inside – all I had to do was turn the dial to the correct dosage, put the end of the pen against my skin then depress the end. I'd hear a short click and the needle would shoot out into my skin, delivering the right amount of drug. Apparently, the place with least pain involved would be my stomach and the advice was to grab a piece of tummy between my fingers, clean it with a sterile swab, rub it with an ice cube, then click. So, really easy then!

I sat in the kitchen watching the clock, with the pen on the table and the swab in my hand, thinking I really should just get on with it. Every second sat watching and putting it off would only make it worse, so I just went into autopilot and did it. One click. Finished. But hey, hang on. It was supposed to hurt wasn't it? I mean, really hurt. All I had was a small pin prick and scratch, and a bit of stinging when the drug went in. I was really rather pleased with myself – it wasn't as bad as I'd thought. I got up, put the swabs and cotton wool away in their box, and the injection pen back in the fridge. And that was what I did for the next seven days.

Friday, 12th August 2005
The week went by quite quickly and it was soon time for my ultrasound scan and blood test. I made the now familiar trip to the hospital as usual, then went home to wait until 3.10 p.m., when I had to phone in to get my results. At this point I could think of nothing else but the impending procedure. Would I be ready for egg collection?

Which day would it be? When would the transfer take place afterwards?

The rest of the morning and early afternoon went by so slowly it was like watching paint dry. I suppose it was because everything was all so new and unknown – unexplored territory if you like. I called my mum for a chat – she was going to come down and stay for a few days, and would be in the room with me when I had my eggs collected. James had planned to be, but the thought of it made him feel rather ill, and he was quite happy for my mum to be there instead. I told her I wouldn't know until later that day what the plan was – it wasn't easy making arrangements as she still worked and had to take some days off or rearrange with a colleague, without anyone else knowing why.

3.10 p.m. came around and I telephoned the unit. The nurse told me that I wouldn't be going in for egg collection on Monday as I 'wasn't quite ready yet'. My spirits dipped. I knew it didn't mean anything really, just that they wanted my follicles to mature to have the opportunity of retrieving more and/or better eggs. Still, I couldn't help but be disappointed. I'd really geared myself up for Monday morning so I felt a bit deflated. That feeling of not being in control surfaced again too – I was completely at the beck and call of people who didn't have any emotional attachment to what we were going through whatsoever.

Monday, 15th August 2005
One final scan and blood test later the date for egg collection was confirmed as Wednesday, 17th August and I was given instructions on when to do my late-night shot of booster

hormone, my last injection before egg collection day. This is a hormone which mimics one that is produced naturally, LH (luteinising hormone), resulting in the rupture of the follicles and subsequent release of eggs. It was absolutely vital that I administered the injection exactly as advised, as the egg collection was timed with such precision as to maximise the quantity of eggs. I was told to do it at 10.45 p.m., so when the time came I jabbed my abdomen with the final shot, put the kettle on for a cup of tea then tried to relax for a while before going to bed around midnight. As I drifted off to sleep my thoughts turned to what was to come. One door in the process had closed, and another started to open. My head was heavy but my heart was hopeful. I actually managed to get some rest, and planned to enjoy my one day free of anything medical, before focusing on egg collection day.

Tuesday, 16th August 2005
Well, that had been the plan anyway! My head didn't let me relax much though, as my thoughts were constantly about the next unknown. I couldn't settle or concentrate on anything. I felt as if I was in limbo, just floating around waiting for the next day. I thought to myself that I'd better try and get a sense of calm from somewhere – if I was like this now, then I would have gone completely mad by the end of the two weeks after the egg collection, when I had to wait to find out if I was pregnant or not.

My mum arrived in the morning and we just spent the day in town in an attempt to distract me. She kept asking if I was getting nervous, and told me I was brave, but I said I wasn't either of those things. I didn't want her to worry and quite successfully managed to cover up any anxieties that were creeping up on me. I knew that really I was starting to get nervous, even though the procedure was classed as being minor. I'd read many stories from women who'd experienced a lot of pain during and after the egg collection and had concluded that I would feel the same. I kept trying to think positively, even though no thinking in the world would alter the outcome, or my experience. I knew that focus and concentration could go some way to easing or blocking a lot of potential physical pain, but as my mind raced I found it incredibly difficult to zone out and find that calm place in my head. I'd read about trying to envisage a desert island or somewhere, but I just couldn't still my thoughts enough to do it.

By late evening I decided to go to bed – if I managed to fall asleep straight away it could give me the space I needed. We had to be up early in the morning anyway as the egg collection was planned for 9.45 a.m., which meant we'd be travelling to the hospital in Oxford's rush hour. I wanted to leave the house at 8.45 a.m., giving plenty of time for what was normally a twenty minute journey – there was no way I wanted to risk getting stressed about being caught in traffic.

Wednesday, 17th August 2005

Egg collection day dawned and we set off for the hospital as planned. On arrival we parked in the nearest space we could find – like most hospital car parks, spaces were like gold dust so if you saw one you nabbed it, and fast.

Once in the unit we sat in the waiting room and I did a mental check of everything I'd had to bring or do – spare pair of knickers for after the procedure, check (bleeding was usual); all nail varnish removed, check (apparently it could affect the embryos so wasn't allowed at all); someone to drive me home afterwards, check.

We didn't have to wait long this time before we were called through, our identities were verified and we were given a consent form to read and sign. The name at the top of the form said 'transvaginal egg collection'. James started to look a bit worried. He read through it and became concerned about the section that stated the 'serious or frequently occurring risks'. The doctor, or nurse, had written 'infection/bleeding/bowel damage'. I must admit I was also a bit worried about it, but the nurse explained that whilst the risks were minimal, lawfully we still had to be informed. It didn't mean that there was any real risk worth noting. I told James that it was quite irrelevant anyway – we'd come this far, and there was no way I was going to back out now, just because of a theoretical risk. I think he knew that too really; it was just unexpected and he was obviously concerned for me.

The procedure meant that I would be sedated, whilst an ultrasound scan was used to guide a fine needle into the ovaries through the muscle of the vaginal wall. Each large fluid filled sac (follicle) should contain an egg, but smaller ones may not. The fluid would then be drained from all visible follicles in both ovaries one by one and the presence of a microscopic egg in the fluid would be confirmed immediately by the embryologist. Depending on the amount of follicles, the procedure would take about forty minutes or so. As I mentioned before we'd already agreed that my mum would be with me during the procedure as

I knew that James would find it difficult, so the plan was for him to wait for us in the next room.

As the nurse came to fetch me I told James I'd see him soon, gave him a quick kiss, then I entered the treatment room ready for the procedure. I can remember it vividly and I can also remember thinking how small it was – no bigger than an average dentist's. I was expecting something more along the lines of a proper theatre – I'd seen that type of thing on TV when I'd watched some programmes on IVF in the past, so to be in a tiny room like this, jam-packed with equipment and several nurses was quite strange. There was also a little hatch to the side, where the fluid from each follicle would be passed through to the embryologist who would confirm whether there was an egg in it. The hatch was lifted up and someone suddenly appeared saying a cheery "hello". It was actually rather comical and I wondered whether she was going to ask me if I wanted a cup of tea! She told me that she was the embryologist and explained what she would be doing, as I'd be completely unaware due to the strong sedation.

I lay down on the bed, hutched my lower half over the end and put my feet in the stirrups. Completely ungainly and zero dignity. It felt a bit humiliating, although I didn't really have much time to dwell on that as the anaesthetist sat next to me and put a cannula in my hand to administer the sedation drugs. Everyone else introduced themselves, my mum was installed on a chair next to me holding my hand, and the next thing I remember was lying on a bed in the next room asking how it had gone. The answer was, "quite well", although I did wonder why everyone seemed to be having a fit of the giggles – apparently I refused to get off the treatment bed into the wheelchair and had to be hauled off by several people. I can't remember it at all; it was obviously a very effective sedative.

The room I'd been transferred to was not particularly comfortable or welcoming – it was like a mini ward with curtains separating three beds, each having all of about a foot of space to the side in which to fit a small chair. It wasn't private at all and I felt like I was on a production line. I was instructed to stay on the bed whilst the drugs wore off and until I was able to stand without toppling over. As some bleeding was expected I'd also been given an absolutely gigantic sanitary pad – hadn't they heard of Bodyform for goodness sake?

I chatted to James and my mum for a while, and listened to everything going on around us as there were several couples in that day for the same procedure. My thoughts at the time were ones of practicality rather than any specific emotions or feelings, but I do recall being thankful that it was all over. After a while a nurse came to see us and told us that they'd retrieved twelve eggs; nine were graded 'good', one 'middle', and two 'not so good' – whatever that meant. We were then told we could go home and I was instructed not to drive or cook for the next forty-eight hours due to the effects of the painkillers. It was a good job my mum had planned on staying for a few days.

As soon as I left the hospital building and got in the car I suddenly felt extremely uncomfortable. I'm not sure whether it was the way I was sat or the angle of the car seat but I felt a bit tight around my middle, and quite sore. I suppose that was to be expected given what I'd just had done; all I wanted to do was go home to rest.

Once back at the apartment, James took a late train and went into work. There was no point in him hanging around for the rest of the day, especially given my mum was with me. It was only lunchtime and he'd at least be able to get something done if he went into the office for a couple of hours. I was completely shattered anyway, and ended up falling asleep on the sofa. By the time I woke up it was early evening, and after some dinner prepared by my mum I found that my eyes just wouldn't stay open.

Thursday, 18th August 2005

Early in the morning I received the promised telephone call telling us that the ICSI procedure had worked, and that I was to go back to the unit on Friday for two embryos to be transferred. I thanked the nurse then put the phone down and told James and my mum what she'd just said. In total we had five successful embryos and my initial reaction was that it was quite a good outcome. I felt really positive that as well as the two we'd be transferring we might have some to freeze. It would cost more for the unit to keep them in storage but it was worth doing if the embryos were of a good enough quality by Friday.

Although we were all really excited by the news and it felt like we'd reached another watershed moment, we were also acutely aware that there was no guarantee that any of them would still be viable by Friday. They had all divided as was to be expected so far though, and whilst I was conscious of not getting too carried away there was every indication that the embryo transfer would go ahead as planned.

The rest of the day turned out to be a very hot one. My mum and I decided to go into Oxford for lunch so I could get some fresh air and try and keep my mind off things. We left the car in a car park near the Botanical Gardens and walked over the bridge and down into the High Street. I was incredibly slow as I'd started to feel quite tight and bloated again, so it took us ages just to walk as far as the indoor market. Once we got there I decided it was far enough though, so we retraced our steps and stopped off for something to eat in a café back towards the way we'd just come. My mum constantly asked if it was a good idea for me to walk around, but I felt that I needed to move a bit to get my circulation going. Obviously, too much exercise at that point would've been strenuous, but I was quite healthy normally so there was no reason to be completely immobile.

We finished our lunch then returned to the car and headed for home. As it was a pleasant day we put up the deckchairs in the communal gardens so we could read for a while. Not that we did – we just ended up talking about life and stuff. Mum asked me how I felt and told me again how brave she thought I was, at which point I wholeheartedly disagreed. She then got a bit ahead of herself by being all excited about the quantity of eggs and subsequent embryos so I reminded her that it was just one hurdle amongst many, and we had to take it one step at a time. I tried not to think about the positive 'what ifs' because if things didn't go well I didn't want to be completely disappointed by getting my hopes up too early on.

In the end we had a nice afternoon just doing nothing, although I started to feel a bit more uncomfortable later on when the soreness began to feel worse. It wasn't bad enough to worry me though and I had no other symptoms apart from slight bloating, so I assumed it was just down to being 'messed around with'. However, by late evening I felt absolutely shattered yet again and once more I fell asleep on the sofa, finally hauling myself off to bed when I awoke a short time later. I really needed to rest so I was ready for the big day on Friday.

Friday, 19th August 2005

Having arrived early at the hospital I'd been allocated a room in the fertility unit where I could have my acupuncture session. A few months earlier I'd read somewhere that acupuncture could improve the success of IVF, and as it wasn't detrimental in any way I thought it was definitely worth giving it a go. I'd found a practitioner through a clinic in Oxford, and although she usually worked from home she was quite happy to meet me at the hospital on this occasion. The plan was to have one session just before embryo transfer, followed by another one directly afterwards.

So, there I was in a small scan room with numerous acupuncture needles in my hands, stomach, ears, feet and legs. I'd never had acupuncture before and during my test session some weeks prior, I'd actually felt quite nervous. However, I now knew what to expect so when a new needle was inserted and I felt a strange 'dragging' sensation, I knew it was working. I had to stay still for around thirty minutes with the needles in position. Occasionally the practitioner moved them slightly, or rotated them, but other than that it was actually quite a pleasant experience.

At around 10.45 a.m. a nurse checked in on us to see if I was about ready for the transfer. The needles were just being removed, so the timing couldn't have been better. I got my things together then my mum and I were shown into the same room that had been used for the egg collection a couple of days ago. James hadn't come as my mum was with me and he'd only have hung around looking like a lemon anyway, so he went to work as normal.

Once in the room we were shown a monitor next to the bed where we were able to see the catheter inserted into my uterus through my cervix, hopefully followed by the embryos in the fluid. It was a very old black and white monitor with what looked like lots of dark spots and grainy areas – obviously we didn't really know what we were looking for, but as the catheter was inserted the nurse pointed it out to us so we'd be able to see the fluid come through the end. After a minute or so the embryologist said that the embryos were in the catheter, then the fluid was released and the catheter was retracted. That was it. Transfer done.

In comparison to the egg collection it was such a quick and simple procedure. I was given some suppositories called Cyclogest containing a hormone that supports implantation, as my own body would not be making enough initially. They were like tampons and I had to insert one each morning and evening for fifteen days. I would find out later that this was quite a messy operation, and it was best to lie down for half an hour straight afterwards!

For the next two weeks I was advised to have a shower rather than a bath, and to avoid swimming until after the pregnancy test. You had to be joking really – why on earth would I want to do any exercise with this precious cargo on board? Anything that could possibly alter the outcome was completely off the agenda for me. Whether that was being paranoid was irrelevant – I had to be sure in my mind that nothing I did would affect anything, so for two weeks it was rest and recuperation, with the occasional slow walk to get some fresh air. Anyway, we'd planned to go away for a long weekend the following Thursday, so that gave me plenty of time in which to do absolutely nothing.

Amongst the other warnings I was given that concerned side effects of both the procedure and the hormonal suppositories, I do remember the print in bold font on the advice sheet that said, *"extreme bloatedness, abdominal swelling or pain, high temperature or breathlessness"*, was a reason to contact the unit. It looked a bit scary, but I didn't really give it much thought to be honest. It said that some women experienced a small amount of brown blood loss for one or two days in the week following embryo transfer, and that this was minimal and should stop after a couple of days. It also said that the drugs (the Cyclogest suppositories), *"may cause side effects that are associated with early pregnancy such as nausea, breast tenderness etc."* then went on to say that, *"this is quite normal"* and, rather callously, that it *"...does not mean that you are pregnant"*. Not only had I suffered the procedure in the first place, I was then tortured with the fact that any pregnancy symptoms could just be phantom ones.

In addition to all the information there was a section that gave me the date I had to do the pregnancy test – Friday, September 2nd 2005. I have no idea how I got through the next two weeks – I was in a constant state of limbo and how I wished I could have forgotten about it for the whole time. To say it had turned into a bit of an obsession was an understatement. I knew I had to try and relax somehow or other. It ended up being the longest two weeks of my life.

After nodding in agreement to everything the nurses told me, and after they'd made sure I was stable enough to walk we were free to go. My mum drove me home and when we were safely back in the apartment she put the kettle on for the obligatory cup of tea. Shortly after, as it was a Friday and she didn't want to get caught in traffic and had to go to work on Saturday, she made me promise to call her if I needed anything, then said goodbye and left. It was the first time after the procedure that I was on my own and as I sat in the living room and tried to distract myself by reading a magazine, my mind wouldn't focus no matter how hard I tried.

After an unexpectedly calm night when I slept right through until morning, we had the whole weekend ahead of us. It turned out to be nothing out of the ordinary and we ended up doing our usual routine – had breakfast, went into Oxford for lunch, visited the bookshops, had coffee, then came home late afternoon. We may have even gone to the cinema, I really can't remember. I do know, however, that we would have had tomato pasta for dinner. We always had that on Saturday – James didn't know which day of the week it was otherwise!

Thursday, 25th August 2005
It was time for our mini holiday – yippee! It was only to Poole and Bournemouth but I'd reserved a room in a

smart boutique hotel, and as we hadn't been anywhere for a couple of years it was really nice just to get away for a few days. We'd been to the Sandbanks area before, so were already familiar with it – one thing we wanted to do was play the crazy golf next to the beach, which is a little bit sad and incredibly naff! I always lost as I wasn't much good with my aim, but we always had a laugh and it was something we just didn't do very often. I suppose it was a throwback to our childhood – I could remember playing it in Skegness when we went on day trips when I was little – not sure about James's excuse though.

It was nearly a week since the transfer and so far so good – I felt fairly normal and was quite positive. I'd been really organised and managed to pack everything ready to go and I'd even managed to fit in one last acupuncture session the day before we left. We decided to drive down as it was only a couple of hours away, so we set off from Oxford late morning. We hadn't gone far though when we stopped at the Newbury services to have something to eat and a cup of tea – all of about twenty minutes' drive.

We found a table then sat down and began to eat in between chatting about this and that. There were a couple of small children in highchairs near us, and we both noticed them at the same time. We just looked at each other as if to say, "that could be us soon", but not quite daring to speak the words – a rather awkward moment that passed as quickly as it came.

We arrived at our destination mid-afternoon. It was a contemporary hotel with great views, although our room was a big disappointment. It was tiny and impossible to get round the bed to the bathroom without having to walk sideways – the end of it nearly reached right up to the wall. We thought it was rather odd; that it looked like they'd squeezed an extra double room in when really it shouldn't have been built there. We didn't mention it though as there would've been no point. They wouldn't have moved us as, being August, the hotel was fully booked, and as we planned to be out most of the time it didn't really matter anyway.

We explored the rest of the hotel then wandered down to the bar where we ordered tea and coffee. We decided to eat at the hotel that night as we really couldn't be bothered to go anywhere else seeing as I was quite tired, again. We asked for a table at the restaurant and were surprised to find that they couldn't fit us in – apparently they'd booked some tables for non-residents. I was a bit cross that no-one had thought to ask us at the time of booking whether we wanted to reserve a table in the restaurant. OK, so maybe we should have thought of that ourselves too, but just a bit of initiative on their part might have been nice.

We thought about what to do for a moment then I remembered a little Italian place in Bournemouth near the gardens – Valentino's. It was run by an Italian guy, so it was proper authentic food. It was still early evening so we knew we'd have no problem getting in if we left straight away.

We arrived in Bournemouth and parked the car just down the road near the gardens. We got to the restaurant really early, about 6.30 p.m. I think, so we managed to get a decent table. As we waited James asked me how I was. I made a point of saying that I felt absolutely fine and any soreness I'd had from the previous week had disappeared.

I was still counting down the days of the two week wait, but that was to be expected and overall I was quite encouraged.

We both ordered garlic bread to start, then James had a pizza and I had lasagne. I remembered this restaurant so well because the food really was good, and it always arrived piping hot – steaming to be precise. The first time we ate there several years before I'd burnt the roof of my mouth off. The chef did warn us, but it was still a bit unexpected – it obviously didn't put us off though.

After we'd finished our main meals there was just no room left for any more food, so we skipped pudding. I didn't think anything of it at the time, but my stomach suddenly started to feel uncomfortably tight – it felt as if someone had pumped a tyre up inside me. I just put it down to heavy pasta with all that melted cheese, so we decided to have a tea or coffee in our room, rather than stay for cappuccino (not that I was drinking caffeine of course). I commented to James on the way back that I was completely 'stuffed', and all I wanted to do was unzip my trousers and let my waist expand. I hoped the feeling would have disappeared by morning.

Friday, 26th August 2005

And so it did. Except it'd been replaced by a different, stranger sensation. I can't describe it really. I just didn't feel 'right'. I didn't have a headache. My stomach wasn't bloated, tight, or painful and I didn't feel nauseous; I was just a bit hot and unsettled. It had been a bit warm all night; not outside, but the room felt stifling. I mentioned it to James and he didn't seem to think it was overly hot. Maybe it was just me and I'd had a reaction to the pessaries.

I put it to the back of my mind and we set out for Poole.

It didn't take us long to get to town. We parked in the multi-storey belonging to the shopping centre, then made our way slowly down to the harbour through the main shopping zone, stopping on the way occasionally to browse. There were several games shops that James was interested in, and a couple of little independent upmarket gift ones that I liked. After a short walk we arrived at the quay. To say it was August there wasn't really that much going on and it was very quiet. Mind you the weather wasn't exactly fantastic – it was bank holiday weekend so inevitably it was raining!

We looked at the information about boat excursions and saw that one was due to leave for a round-trip around Brownsea Island, just outside the harbour. It only took about an hour so we bought a couple of tickets then boarded and sat on the open-air top level. It was surprisingly full, but once it stopped at Brownsea Island almost everyone got off. The weather started to change a bit too and I became quite cold, so we decided to go and sit downstairs in the bar area – not that it was open in the middle of the day.

I sat down on the banquette style chairs and looked around. It wasn't actually that nice – definitely more of a ferry than anything resembling luxury. The seats were covered in a blue plastic-like material, and many of them were ripped. The boat had a tinny sound to it, and was devoid of any atmosphere. It felt like we were out of season rather than at the end of August. We still had half an hour or so to go though so I just enjoyed the views and listened to the commentary about the history of the island and Old Harry Rocks.

After a few minutes had passed I suddenly became aware of the motion of the boat and mentioned to James that I began to feel a bit odd – a bit nauseous. I lay down on a banquette and tried to centre myself to counteract the movement. It didn't work though and I just wanted to get off. I did have a tendency towards car sickness, and I had a bad experience on a ferry to France once, so I really didn't think anything of it, other than wanting to have my feet on solid ground.

Before long we arrived back at the quay and disembarked as quickly as possible. I still felt queasy and needed to walk a bit to get my circulation going again. We looked in a few more shops then decided to go and get some lunch. Once back in the main shopping area we found a little café that served simple food like traditional salads and sandwiches. We didn't need to fill up too much anyway as we had our table booked at the hotel restaurant that night. I was incredibly thirsty too so James ordered several bottles of water for me.

After a quick look round the indoor shopping centre we decided to go back to the hotel to rest or read for a while. I still felt strange – not to the point of worried, but it definitely wasn't normal. I knew my body well and it was trying to tell me something, although quite what I wasn't sure at that point.

We found the pedestrian entrance to the car park and opted to take the stairs back to our level as the lift was quite busy. James walked ahead a bit as we couldn't remember exactly where the stairs were, so he'd gone off to investigate. I spotted him waiting at the end of the corridor and when I caught up with him I must have looked a bit strange because he asked me if I was OK. I waved him on and said, "I think so, I just suddenly feel a bit breathless," so he started off up the stairs. I put one foot in front of the other to go up behind him, but found that I couldn't do it. I called out to him that I didn't know why, but I couldn't get up the stairs. It was like I couldn't get enough oxygen to my lungs and it really felt as though I was overexerting myself. I looked at James in a slight panic. I didn't know what was wrong and I started to get a bit frightened, although I didn't say so as he looked a bit irritated that I'd changed my mind about the stairs. He came back down and we walked over to the lift. I told him I felt breathless and I just didn't feel right. I could see that he'd started to get a bit concerned, and he asked me again if I was alright. I just kept saying, "I think so," over and over again. I didn't know otherwise; I hadn't experienced anything like it before.

I tried not to think about it as we got in the car. It was OK. I'd begun to breathe normally again. I drank some water and looked out of the window, trying to convince myself that it was just the procedure and tiredness catching up with me.

Once back at the hotel we spent the rest of the day just relaxing, then headed downstairs to the restaurant. We were seated at a table facing the terrace so I was able to look out at the view. As James busied himself with the wine list I decided what to order – there was a lot to choose from and it took me ages to decide. I can't remember what I ate, but it was definitely delicious and my dress slowly felt tighter and tighter as the evening went on. "Too much food again", I thought, or rather was hoping that was what it was. It wasn't too unpleasant though and I wasn't out of breath, although it would've really taken something quite serious to do that whilst sitting down!

We finished the meal off with coffee or in my case a peppermint tea, then went back to our room. It was actually quite tiring just being near the sea and not doing much, and after an hour or so of reading I was ready for sleep.

Saturday, 27ᵗʰ August 2005

Saturday dawned and I felt a little better so we decided to go into Bournemouth. During the drive I called the fertility unit in Oxford to let them know I'd had some symptoms, just in case. I dialled the number on the after-care advice sheet and asked to speak to any available doctor. As it was Saturday and a bank holiday weekend I wasn't even sure if anyone would be there, but luckily I managed to speak to one of the female doctors. I explained my symptoms and she told me not to worry and that it was probably just my body recovering. As I was able to move around she thought it wasn't necessary to do anything else except try and stay hydrated and to call back if anything developed. I was glad that it all sounded normal to her, and it did ease my mind a little so I tried to forget about it and just enjoy myself.

After we parked the car and walked down to the gardens we saw that there were several events going on and there was quite a crowd, so we found some deckchairs near the bandstand, away from the main activity area. It was quite pleasant but I got bored really quickly, and whilst James had some books from work with him I had nothing with me, so I went for a walk into the town and left James to his mathematical equations or whatever. There would be far more interesting things to see in the local boutiques.

I spent the next hour or so just browsing. I went into a couple of department stores and found it really difficult not to go to the baby and children's section. I didn't want to tempt fate – not that I believed just looking would make any difference to the outcome, but my superstitious irrational self told me not to even think about it at that point. It was difficult though – it was the first time I'd been alone in a while and so far I'd managed to temper my thoughts to a certain degree, but as soon as I was on my own my mind started to go over things again and again.

I decided to go back to James in the gardens to see if he wanted to go in search of ice cream. I found him in exactly the same position as when I'd left with his pile of books next to the deckchair, and gave him some grief about being a boring old fart by bringing his work with him, and asked if we could, "Please go and get an ice cream or something?" Although that wasn't such a good plan actually, as once we'd found the Mr Whippy van I decided that it really wasn't wise in my condition – what if it made me ill? I was sure that you should avoid ice cream when pregnant as it contained raw eggs and I could get food poisoning…damn, I was so looking forward to a mint choc chip. James was not amused either.

By this time it was late afternoon and we began to think about where to eat that evening. We'd been to several places earlier in the day to try and book a table, but everywhere was full. We went back to the hotel and asked the receptionist for any ideas. He recommended a hotel down the hill which probably had some available tables. We phoned and managed to get in for around 8 p.m., so after a short nap and freshen up we set off.

It was about a fifteen minute walk and as it was a warm evening it was really pleasant. The hotel was situated right on the beach and was very large and busy. I was glad that we hadn't booked to stay there – I preferred smaller hotels usually. There were too many people, and after seeing the dining room it felt a bit like a factory. We sat down and placed our order with the waiter. James said he didn't feel like eating much, but to be honest I think the atmosphere just put him off completely. I agreed that it wasn't really our thing, but as we'd ordered already we had to stay. We ate our soup then waited for the main course to arrive. In the meantime I began to feel a bit odd – sort of 'squashed'. It was weird, but after two mouthfuls of main course my stomach felt as if it had expanded a hundredfold and I just couldn't eat any more. I told James and he seemed a bit cross that I'd ordered and wasn't going to eat it but it was really unexpected, and completely unlike me not to finish a meal when we were out.

My breathing started to feel slightly laboured too, so I asked James if we could go back to our hotel as I needed to lie down. He paid the bill and we left at around 9 p.m. It was an uphill walk on the way back so I took my shoes off as I had high heels on. There was no way I would've made it back wearing them, huffing and puffing like an eighty-year-old chain smoker. James told me not to be daft and that I couldn't walk on the pavement without shoes. I said, "Why not? It's only shoes." If I couldn't walk without them on then he had to carry me back up the hill, at which point he came to his senses and just let me get on with it. It did take ages though as I had to keep stopping for breath and James kept calling out to me to watch out for the dog poo!

Half way up the hill though I started to get a little worried. It clearly wasn't normal and I was really struggling to walk. It felt like the longest journey ever. Once back at the hotel I had to sit in the lobby for a moment or two to try and get my breath. I finally recovered and managed to make it to our room where I flopped on the bed and just looked at the ceiling. My bloated belly was still a bit of a cause for concern although my head told me that some bloating was to be expected – it said so on all the literature I'd been given. I carried on choosing to believe that I was just being unlucky with the other symptoms, and after a good night's sleep all would be fine again in the morning.

Sunday, 28th August 2005

Except I didn't get a good night's sleep. At all. I couldn't get to sleep properly in the first place. Whichever way I turned it was uncomfortable – it felt as if I was lying on a rubber ring. I tossed and turned for ages, and I knew I'd disturbed James. I was also really thirsty, and had to keep getting up to go to the bathroom for a pee, except I couldn't 'go'. It felt like cystitis yet it wasn't. The whole night went by very slowly and when morning finally came around I was so tired. After what felt like the hundredth time of trying to pee I said to James that I thought we should go home. We hadn't been due to return until Monday, but I felt really unwell and knew that I wouldn't want to do anything 'touristy'. He immediately agreed – there was no point in staying as we'd have just ended up in our hotel room with me pacing the floor; I needed the comforts of home. James rang down to reception and advised them that we had to leave early as I wasn't feeling well. They came up to collect our luggage and after we checked out James loaded up the car with the bags and we began the drive home.

I thought it might be wise to call the fertility unit again so I dialled the emergency number that I'd rung the previous day. I managed to get through and spoke to someone who took my details then told me that my consultant would call back shortly. James started to get a little worried so we decided to just drive straight back home without stopping for a break. I put my head on the back of the seat and tried to centre myself. I needed to empty my mind so I could relax, but I was unable to ignore my thoughts.

After an hour or so my mobile rang; it was my consultant, Mr Child. He asked me to explain my symptoms so I told him everything that had happened since Thursday. He said that although it sounded nothing to worry about it was probably a good idea to get to the hospital so I could be checked out. I told him we were on route back from our holiday and it would take us a couple of hours to get to there, at which point he explained that we were to go directly to the fertility unit where someone would be 'on call' and he'd let them know we were on our way. I ended the conversation and told James what Mr Child had said. We decided to go back home first to drop off the bags and an hour and a half later we pulled into the driveway. James took all the bags inside then got straight back in the car to take me to the hospital.

As it was a Sunday the roads were fairly quiet and it only took us fifteen minutes or so to get there. We made our way up to the unit and were then redirected to one of the women's wards on the ground floor where they were expecting us. After giving our details we were asked to wait so I sat on a chair in the corridor and closed my eyes. I wasn't exactly panicking but I was quite concerned – I was hot and heavy and still felt nauseous, and the feeling of tiredness was overwhelming.

Forty-five minutes or so later we were ushered into a side consulting room, where a nurse asked me about my symptoms again. She made some notes then left the room, saying that the doctor would be in shortly to take a look at me. By this time I was feeling quite flushed, still very hot and a bit dizzy. It was obvious to me now that something definitely wasn't right, and I told James that I thought the treatment hadn't worked.

The doctor finally arrived and asked me to sit on the bed, then took all the details yet again. He looked at my records from the fertility unit then told me that he thought there was nothing to worry about. It looked like I'd just had a strong reaction to the treatment procedure and my bloated stomach, whilst a little tight, was considered mild. He advised me to go home, make sure I rested and just monitor how I felt. If the symptoms got worse I had to call back. Overall he was very matter-of-fact about it. I assumed he'd obviously seen it all before, and he did put my mind at rest – I'd seen someone at the hospital, had been checked over, and nobody was alarmed by anything. The thought of feeling like this overnight again wasn't exactly great, but as I was so tired maybe I'd just fall asleep really quickly and have a restful night.

We got back in the car and went home, stopping on the way at the petrol station supermarket to pick up something to eat, given it was Sunday and the shops were closed. I put the radio on in the car and we joked a bit about how daft we were and that everything would be fine. I was ten days into my two week wait and a tiny glimmer of hope appeared.

Monday, 29th August 2005

I must have been exhausted as I managed to sleep through finally, and I lay awake but dozing for a while. It was around 9 a.m. when I needed to go to the bathroom so I swung my legs round the side of the bed and shuffled into the ensuite. I felt a bit peculiar, as if I'd been up all night, so I knew I wasn't any better. I just hoped I wasn't any worse. I got up to flush the loo when I suddenly went very hot and clammy. I felt really dizzy and sat straight back down again as a wave of nausea came over me and the room began to swim in front of my eyes. I was going to faint and all I could think about was James finding me on the floor after I'd blacked out and smacked my head against the shower door on the way down. Survival instinct or something must have kicked in at that point as I became completely focused on remaining calm. I tried not to panic, and after a couple of minutes had passed made myself get up very slowly.

I reached the bathroom door then tentatively walked back into the bedroom where I sat on the edge of the bed, closed my eyes and tried to stop the room from moving. I told James what had just happened and that he had to ring the hospital straight away. I think he could tell by the look on my face that I was completely serious, and that something must really be wrong for me to suggest calling the hospital.

I just sat there trying to steady myself as he dialled the now familiar number. He hastily explained everything to the nurse, and we were told to pack a bag and get there as soon as possible. James pulled a holdall out of the wardrobe and started to pack it for me. I couldn't think straight. What would I need? Pyjamas and a toothbrush obviously, but what about anything else? We decided just to take the basics. If I ended up staying in overnight for observation then James could always come home and get some more things for me; it wasn't as if we were miles away.

We slowly made our way down the stairs of our apartment building. I had to grab the handrail as I found it quite difficult just to put one foot in front of the other – the rate at which the dizziness took hold was dismaying. I finally made it down the stairs and into the car, and we drove to the hospital in silence. I think James really didn't know what to say, and I just didn't want to say what I knew. I tried to put it out of my mind – this was just a setback; I'd be fine. For some reason I'd had a bad reaction, but that didn't mean the treatment hadn't worked – as yet I still hadn't had a bleed and it was now Monday, ten days after the transfer. That was a good sign. Wasn't it?

We arrived at the hospital, parked the car, and made our way to the women's gynaecology ward. We checked in at the reception then were told to sit and wait and someone would come to fetch us. No sooner had I sat down than a nurse came over and led us to the same room we'd been in the previous day. Shortly after that a doctor arrived, measured my blood pressure then told us that I had to be admitted to the hospital. I was suffering from a condition called Ovarian Hyperstimulation Syndrome (OHSS).

Chapter 4

The End...?

OHSS was something that had been mentioned in the risks and complications section of the IVF literature. I'd read it before going through the treatment but didn't really pay too much attention as I didn't think it would affect me, as you don't. The information sheet from the hospital said:

The next most frequently encountered risk associated with IVF treatment cycles is that of Ovarian Hyperstimulation Syndrome (OHSS). This complication results from the high hormone levels achieved during super-ovulation (a high number of follicles developing in the ovaries) and affects 2% of all treatment cycles. In OHSS the woman may suffer from abdominal swelling or bloating and feel very tired, thirsty and breathless. Ultrasound scanning of the developing follicles are designed to minimise this risk, but occasionally it is necessary to admit the woman to hospital for a few days rest and observation. If OHSS symptoms are very severe it is sometimes. necessary to abandon the treatment cycle and recommence the cycle at a later date at a lower dose of stimulation.

Now to my mind, that meant that once I'd passed the stage of stimulation and had the egg collection, there would no longer be a risk of it happening. That's why it didn't really enter my head when I started to get symptoms such as tiredness and difficulty breathing – I just assumed that the information I'd been given in the hospital literature was as described and nothing more – why would I question it? They were the experts after all and there was no reason for me to query what had been written.

After hearing what the doctor said, my head tried to process both the diagnosis and the fact that I had to stay in hospital for a while. He told us that it would probably be at least a few days as they wanted to keep their eye on me. Given there was no treatment for OHSS, only management of the symptoms, there was nothing they could do to prevent anything else from happening – they simply had to be there to react 'just in case'.

"Oh", I thought, and went very quiet. I really didn't like spending time in hospitals – I absolutely hated to be away from home unless I was on holiday. My introverted nature meant that the thought of being in hospital, in a ward with people I didn't know and was probably going to have to be sociable with, made me feel completely sick all over again. I started to worry and could feel it in the pit of my stomach. Not only did I have to deal with the uncertainty of my physical self, I was also going to be put in, what was for me, a very stressful environment.

But, there I was, facing the emotional trauma of OHSS and potential non-motherhood at the same time. I looked at the doctor who'd just finished entering some information on my admissions sheet. He signed the form then looked at me and casually said that he was going to put me in my own room. He said that it wasn't appropriate for me to be with the other patients due to my 'condition'. Not only was it a delicate subject, having just had IVF, I would require lots of blood tests, observations, new drips etc., which had potential to disrupt the ward too much and he'd decided that a separate room would be best.

Well, he must have read my mind. The relief of not having to be in a ward was immeasurable. It might seem a bit trivial given the circumstances, but to have been given my own space so that I could just be with myself and my thoughts, able to read (or worry) in peace undisturbed, or just to do nothing without hearing other people's conversations, would make a huge difference to my state of mind. I thanked the doctor, who said it was the least they could do. He then confirmed that the room was already available and I could go straight in. He led us out of the consultation room, round by the nurses' station, past a ward on the left and to a small corridor at the end, where he showed us into my room. It was situated next to another single room, with a shared toilet and bathroom/shower cubicle just outside the door.

I sat on the bed and the nurse asked me to get into my nightdress (pyjamas were, apparently, too uncomfortable, given their expectation of what was about to happen...), and that she would be back to insert a cannula to hook me up to a drip to try to rehydrate me as quickly as they could. The reason I'd nearly passed out in the bathroom at home was because of severe dehydration, and it had to be reversed as soon as possible.

I watched James as he unpacked the few things I'd

brought, then I asked him if he'd call my parents. I didn't want to do it myself – I knew that my mum would be incredibly worried, and as I was already rather emotional I didn't think I'd be able to stop myself from getting too upset. It was easier anyway – James was going home to collect some more things for me – books, music, decent food and snacks etc. It would give him chance to call my mum and dad, and for me to settle in a bit and contemplate my situation.

After a couple of minutes a nurse returned with all the equipment for the drip, and to take some blood. James said he'd wait until they'd hooked me up before he went back home to get everything sorted. I looked at the cardboard tray with the cannula and a syringe on it, still in their wrappings, as the nurse tied a disposable glove round my arm to serve as a tourniquet. I thought that was a rather novel use of a disposable glove, and one I'd not seen before. I'd heard that the NHS often had funding issues, but that was taking it a bit far really!

Anyway, after some deliberation, the nurse decided to insert the cannula into the vein running along the inside of my left wrist, right next to the bone. I wasn't too impressed to say the least – wasn't it supposed to go in the top of your hand? I had visions of it being difficult to move my hand without it hurting once in place – and I was right. Oh well, I didn't say anything. I didn't want them to think I was an upstart by trying to tell them how to do their job – I had to stay there for a few days at least and didn't need the nurses giving me grief.

I looked away when the nurse put the cannula in. Normally I was OK with blood tests and things but I had a preconceived idea that it would hurt when she did it, and if I looked in the other direction I'd be distracted.

As it happened, although it was difficult for her to get it in the right place and she made several attempts, it wasn't too bad. James was rather white though. I'd forgotten that the sight of needles sent him a bit light-headed. The nurse immediately took some blood then said she'd be back later to take some more – it would be at least twice a day, and by the end of my stay all of my 'good' veins had collapsed and I resembled a pin cushion!

By this time it was around 1 p.m. and I was quite hungry. The usual lunch period had just finished but apparently there was some shepherd's pie left if I wanted it. I didn't have a choice really, so I said yes. I'd hardly eaten anything before we left the apartment, and with the events of the morning having been quite draining I needed something in my stomach. This also seemed like a good time for James to go off and get my things, but before disappearing he arranged for the Patientline TV and phone to be activated, so at least I wouldn't go too crazy during my stay. It was also internet enabled so I could check my emails and do some research about my condition, which ended up not being a particularly good idea. A nurse then arrived with my lunch, so James kissed me goodbye and said he'd see me in a couple of hours.

I sat on my bed and got to work on my shepherd's pie. Not bad really, given it was hospital food. There was also some cheese and biscuits so I polished those off too. I sat for a while and tried to empty my head of everything whizzing round it. It was hard though – the more I tried the more the questions kept popping up. I concentrated so much on not thinking that I started to get a really bad headache. I looked around the room. There was a basin in the corner, a tall side table to the right of my bed, a chair in the other corner and a smaller cabinet to my left. There was also one of those mobile tables on wheels. That was it – very basic, very functional. At least I had plenty of daylight though, as the room had a large double window that overlooked the grounds and an inner courtyard.

I closed my eyes and tried to rest for a while but was soon disturbed by the telephone. I picked it up straight away and heard my mum's voice on the other end. As predicted she was a bit panicky and upset. She said they'd already packed their bags and would arrive in a couple of hours. I knew she'd want to come down and to be honest I was glad. I really didn't want to be completely alone and as James had a lot of work to do he was only able to visit in the evenings. I knew my mum and dad would come to see me during the day, the thought of which helped me through the times I was on my own.

We finished our conversation and my mum rang off so they could get on their way. In the meantime a nurse popped in to give me a heparin injection to thin my blood as my pressure was quite low and they needed to make sure I wouldn't get a blood clot, what with being fairly immobile. She mentioned that it may sting a little then rubbed my arm with the swab and inserted the needle. Bloody hell, that was most definitely an understatement; it really hurt! It wasn't so much the needle itself but the solution straight afterwards. I had to have them daily too, and didn't look forward to them at all.

As well as the drip and drugs I had to wear compression stockings, as it was expected that I'd get very bloated and my legs, as well as my abdomen, would balloon. The nurse sat on the end of the bed and began to roll up some seriously grandma-looking long white socks, then made an attempt to put them on my legs. After a bit of a struggle she finally managed it, then disappeared again after saying she'd be back later to do 'obs'.

I daydreamed out of the window for a while thinking about what had happened, still finding it all rather surreal that I was there in hospital with something that I wasn't even at risk to get in the first place – it was hard to get my head around it and I kept trying to figure out, "Why me?" I was still quite light-headed and weak, and doing anything was an effort. I found it very difficult to get up and felt as if I'd been knocked out. My abdomen was like a balloon, I was very pale, and I was constantly exhausted. My head started to hurt again with all the thinking so I lay down and tried to sleep. It was difficult as it was daytime and the sun was streaming in through the window, but at least I could close the door and be by myself.

A little while later I heard a soft knock on the door and my mum's head appeared round the side. I knew I hadn't been sleeping very heavily but I'd probably been dozing as I glanced at the clock and saw that it was late afternoon already. My mum and dad gave me a hug. You could see the worry on my mum's face quite easily – she'd never been able to conceal how she felt. She sat on the edge of the bed and my dad pulled up a chair – we chatted for a while about what the doctors had said and done so far, and I tried to reassure them that it was all just precautionary, and that it was because I'd become so dehydrated and nearly fainted that they wanted to keep an eye on me.

Not long after, James came back with my things – he'd

also nipped into to Marks and Spencer and got me some prepared fruit and grapes, a pile of magazines, and some other bits and bobs he thought I might like. It was difficult to talk about anything but what had happened and how surprising it was – we all felt a bit like it wasn't real and it was strange to be sat in a hospital room at a time when we should have been thinking of the exciting future. On the one hand, everything might still be OK and it was possible that I'd have a positive result on Friday, when I was due to take the pregnancy test. On the other hand, the empty feeling I had inside told me that no matter how much I really tried to be positive and convince myself I would be pregnant, something in my heart knew that this wasn't going to be our time. I so hoped I was wrong. It didn't happen often but on several occasions I'd been so sure of something that had turned out not to be, that it was completely possible my emotions had got the better of me. We had another three days and four nights to go, and it proved to be an awfully long, drawn out wait.

My parents and James suggested that they let me get some rest as it had been a very eventful day. My mum and dad needed to do the same after their drive, and they hadn't eaten yet either. We said our goodbyes and they promised to return as soon as they were allowed the following day. I felt myself getting upset that they had to leave, although I didn't show it. I had to be strong; I knew that my mum would've just worried like mad so I fought back my tears and looked forward to seeing them the next day.

I looked at my pile of books with the aim of taking my mind somewhere else for a while. I picked one and started to read, but just as I was getting into it my phone rang. I answered and was happy to hear my friend, Anna; James must have called her earlier on. She also lived in Oxfordshire with her husband; we'd worked together for a while a couple of years before, and had stayed friends ever since. Now I had to explain why I was in hospital, so I took a deep breath and told her everything.

Tuesday, 30th August 2005
I didn't sleep much overnight. I found the bed really uncomfortable as my abdomen wasn't getting any smaller and whenever I tried to lie on either side it was really painful and difficult to breathe. It was also weird to be in hospital overnight – the last time I'd been an inpatient was when I had a minor operation about ten years ago, and even then it was only during daylight hours. The sound of the nurses walking up and down, then being interrupted every few hours for a damn blood test was incredibly annoying too. I finally managed to nod off around 6 a.m. or so, then a couple of hours later the catering ladies arrived to sort out breakfast. I think they took pity on me as mine was brought to my room when everyone else had to go to the central lounge area and eat theirs at the communal table.

After cornflakes I had some toast, then really, really weak tea, which was appalling but better than nothing. I was given a sheet to fill in for that day's lunch and dinner options – initially it was a bit of a novelty, but after twenty-four hours I came to the conclusion that the food was dreadful and just ended up ordering cheese and crackers followed by jelly. James had promised to bring in some edible food anyway, but at that moment how I longed for a Pot Noodle sandwich (I know, a truly awful habit I'd picked up from goodness knows where, but you couldn't beat a Pot Noodle sandwich for comfort in times of stress!).

I hauled myself out of bed to have a wash and brush my teeth. The cleaners came in to change my bed so I decided to have a shower while I was waiting. I checked the bathroom next door was free then grabbed a towel and my dressing gown and stood under the warm water for five minutes or so. I felt a lot better – almost normal. After drying myself and putting my nightdress back on I sat on my bed. It was only 9 a.m.

My only option was to read again, so I picked up my book and tried to concentrate but my mind kept wandering and I struggled to focus on the characters so I just closed my eyes instead. A nurse came in to take the usual bloods at which point she told me that a doctor would stop by to do observations and check how I was. I smiled and thanked her for letting me know then twiddled my thumbs for a bit whilst I thought about what to do next.

It suddenly dawned on me that I had to phone my work colleague, Ali. As it'd been a bank holiday the day before James had only been able to contact her at home, so I had to give her an update and let my managers know. After a couple of rings she picked up and I explained that I'd be off sick for a few days. She sounded really concerned and said that she'd come down to the hospital during visiting hours to see me. I told her I'd see her later then put the phone down and picked up one of the magazines that James had brought for me.

I was in the middle of an article in *Marie Claire* when my fertility doctor, Mr Child, knocked on the door. He began by saying that it was rather unfortunate to be seeing me again so soon and under these circumstances, and that he'd come by to do a couple of checks to see whether my condition had improved or not. I asked him why he thought my body had reacted as it did, and he said that he was surprised, as I didn't have any of the risk factors normally associated with OHSS. It looked as though I'd just been very, very unlucky.

He examined my abdomen, which was rather uncomfortable as he had to press down quite a lot to gauge what was going on in there, then looked at my charts from the previous day and asked me a couple of questions about how I felt. I told him that I was very uncomfortable, that it felt like I had a weight on my chest, and that I was constantly thirsty. I also found it difficult to walk far as I started to get out of breath, and I hadn't been to the bathroom in ages. He wrote a few things down, then explained what was going to happen.

The reason I found my abdomen tight and heavy was because fluid had leaked from my blood vessels into my body, building up into my chest area. It was making me very dehydrated, and when I did manage to pee it was highly concentrated. The result was that I had to be put on an albumin drip to attempt rehydration and avoid any further action such as paracentesis (a needle inserted into the chest to drain the fluid). I was also to be measured in several places a couple of times per day to check on the build-up, have my urine output calculated every time I went to the bathroom and I had to continually wear the compression stockings on my legs to prevent a blood clot. Drugs-wise it was codeine and twice daily heparin injections. And that was it; then we had to wait. There was nothing else they could do to treat me, it was just a case of managing any symptoms I had and waiting for them to pass.

Well that was just great; I was completely frightened out of my wits. I had visions of something really terrible happening; of having kidney failure or my chest compressing my heart and lungs. I was quite resilient usually, but this just really got to me. Whether it was because of all the emotions involved in the IVF process already, followed by this, or whether it was just because I couldn't cope with not being in control yet again I don't know, but, once my doctor had gone and I was on my own again I couldn't help myself and I just put my head on the pillow and cried. My head hurt, I was confused and I was frightened of the unknown, and, worst of all, I was afraid that the IVF treatment hadn't worked.

I remained still for a while trying to empty my mind, if only to relieve the tension headache that was building. I knew there was absolutely nothing anyone could do and I just had to be patient and get through it. I heard a soft knock on the door again, and a nurse appeared with the drip and lovely fresh white stockings. Perfect; not only did I look like an elephant I was to be encased in something that would make my legs resemble pork sausages and feel like they were cutting off all circulation.

The drip was attached to my arm and a bag of clear fluid clipped into the holder, then the nurse helped me into the stockings. As she turned to leave, my colleague, Ali, turned up with a lovely bouquet of flowers in her arms. She found a vase in the cupboard and arranged them for me then sat down, looked at me with her serious face on, and asked me what the doctors had said.

At that point I knew I had to tell her the real reason I was in hospital. I couldn't sit there face to face with someone I worked with every day and tell her a complete untruth. Or even half a truth – I just had to be honest. Besides, she'd have been able to see if I was being evasive so there was no way I could've given a viable alternative explanation. I found it quite hard saying it though; it felt like failure and embarrassment at the same time.

As I mentioned before, I'm a very private person and often very proud, and thought that I'd be judged if people knew the full story. Still, she was older than me and had her own grown children, so I knew she'd be completely reliable and able to keep it to herself. So I just said it straight out – I told her that we'd been through IVF and I'd had a reaction to the drugs. She said that she'd guessed it was something like that, that it came as no surprise and she wasn't shocked at all. Well, not shocked that we'd had treatment, but she was quite worried about what my body's reaction had been and at my appearance. There I was, all bloated with legs like tree trunks looking completely exhausted with bags and dark circles under my eyes. She just wasn't used to seeing me look so bad and was very concerned. She asked me what I wanted her to say to the rest of my colleagues, although she thought that I should tell them everything. I felt awkward telling them such intimate details of my private life though, given they were male colleagues, and as well as making them feel uncomfortable too I just felt it wasn't necessary to tell them. In the end I asked her to just say as little as possible; something along the lines of I'd had a reaction to some medicine, which was actually the truth.

We chatted a little longer then she returned to work – she'd already taken some extra time to come and see me anyway. We said our goodbyes and she made me promise to call her the moment we had any news on 'testing day'. She closed the door behind her and I was left alone again until my parents arrived a few minutes later.

My mum was anxious when she saw the drip in my arm. I explained to her what it was for and that it was a case of waiting to see how bad the fluid build-up would get. Her face betrayed her thoughts and I could see that she felt completely helpless. Being told to wait and see what happened was difficult to deal with. It was completely out of our hands and we just had to trust the doctors that the albumin drip would work.

To try and lighten the mood I told my mum and dad that I had to take a papier-mâché bedpan with me every time I went to the bathroom, and leave it in there with a paper towel over the top for the nurse to fetch so my urine could be measured! Any remaining vestiges of dignity I had left after the IVF treatment went straight out of the window. The fact that my abdomen had to be measured and charted as well was a double whammy, although from a positive angle at least I'd feel really slim once the bloating had gone down!

My parents stayed for a while longer, but then I really wanted to rest and sleep. My breathing had become shallower by the hour and I felt I needed to try and get in a position that didn't put too much pressure on my chest, which meant half lying down and half sitting up, with the help of several pillows. My eyes were very heavy, and puffy from crying earlier on. I needed to be on my own for a while so that I could get upset in peace and not get anyone else upset at the same time i.e. my parents, especially my mum. I hugged them both then they went off into Oxford for a walk and a coffee. They'd be back next day for another visit before having to return home.

Tuesday night slowly came around and I remained awake wishing away the hours. Sleep was evasive – I couldn't lie on my back at all as it prevented me from breathing. The only position even remotely comfortable was on one side, but after a while I started to get leg ache so I had to swap over, and for some reason I just couldn't settle the other way. My breathing by now was very shallow, it was painful in my chest when I moved position, my legs felt like they had bricks attached, and I was scared. I cried. A lot. Eventually I must have fallen asleep I suppose, but my memory of it was that the night seemed to go on forever.

Wednesday, 31ˢᵗ August 2005

At last it was morning. The nurse came, did my observations and administered more of the dreaded heparin shot. I heard a serving lady from the canteen telling everyone that breakfast was ready then she popped her head round my door and said it was in the rest area if I wanted to go and get it. I managed to ask her before she disappeared if it could be brought to my room. I had no wish whatsoever to sit at a table with people I didn't know when I was feeling so anxious and sick in my stomach from worry. She gave me a withering look that translated as 'lazy cow' – I could see it plainly in her expression and felt awful because next time I knew it'd be an issue. Quite how I was expected to go to the kitchen and fetch a tray of breakfast things then return to my room on my own when I could hardly walk and had a drip attached to my arm was completely beyond me. I suppose it wasn't really their job to think about such things, but as they worked in a hospital a little common sense and empathy would've been nice. It did finally arrive though – cornflakes and a slice of toast. It was all I could eat anyway as my appetite appeared to have gone completely. Or maybe that was just because of the hospital food?

Anyway, after breakfast I was forced up and out of bed as the cleaners did their daily sheets change routine. I took a shower again in the meantime so I wouldn't be hanging around like a spare part, feeling like I was in the way. I grabbed my dressing gown, soap and towel and headed next door to the shower room. I got undressed, looked at the mess that was my body – completely bloated and looking ironically pregnant – then turned on the warm water and just let it run over me. I stood for a minute or so then very quickly started to feel sick and disoriented. I panicked and instinctively pulled the emergency cord. One of the nurses rushed in and asked me if I was alright. I felt as though I was going to fall over so she quickly brought me a chair which allowed me take the weight off my legs, and I just sat there for a couple of minutes. Eventually, after several attempted deep breaths, I seemed to recover and with the help of the nurse managed to dry myself and get back in my nightdress. She suggested that I sit down next time as the fluid in my body meant that I wasn't getting enough oxygen, which was why I'd suddenly felt quite weak and light-headed. My blood pressure was quite low, and moving around wasn't doing me any favours. I realised that I had to be completely bed-bound for the time being, or I'd make everything worse for myself.

It was late morning by the time the doctor came round to see me. He said he was a bit concerned that my urine output was pretty much zero, even though I'd been drinking a lot of fluid. All I was doing was blowing up like a huge balloon and his concern was that they may yet have to do a chest drain, although it was something they really wanted to avoid if at all possible. The decision was to immediately increase the dose of the albumin (protein) drip to see if it would kick-start my system into draining all the fluid. I nodded in agreement; OK, I thought, do what you have to do. I just want to go home.

As expected, the day progressed as if in slow motion. I thought I might watch some morning daytime TV – *Richard and Judy* would be on, or whoever it was that presented it these days. I switched on the television only to be disappointed when I remembered that because it was August the schedule had changed, and it wouldn't be on until the following week when the kids were back at school. Great, I couldn't even watch anything to try and keep me occupied.

I was distracted momentarily by my parents who stopped by again before driving home. My mum really didn't want to leave, but I told her there was no point in staying anyway, as there was nothing anyone could do, and eventually I'd be 'drained' and could go home. I knew she'd phone a couple of times a day to check how I was and have a chat. I heard from James's parents too. I wasn't their daughter so it obviously wasn't as much of a worry but his mum did call me to ask how I was and whether I wanted her to send me a get well card, which made me laugh!

Thursday, 1st September 2005

And so I endured another restless night of punctuated sleep, tossing and turning to try and get comfortable. At one point I really found it difficult to take anything but the slightest gasp of breath and, feeling so completely helpless, I cried yet again for what seemed like ages. My head hurt so much it felt like it was in a vice – briefly remedied by my request for the strongest possible painkillers available.

Morning came around and with it another boring day of staying in bed, reading, eating and trying to sleep. I tried the internet as it was supposedly available through the hospital TV. I attempted to log in but just kept getting an error message when I clicked Internet Explorer, so I called the IT helpline who duly told me that it would take at least twenty-four hours before someone could look at the problem. Why wasn't I surprised?!

By early afternoon I thought there may be something to watch instead, so I skipped through the TV channels and came across *Logan's Run* – a 1970s movie that I could remember from my much younger days. It wasn't exactly top ten cinema material but it took my mind off things for an hour and a half so it served a purpose.

In between all of these exciting activities I'd started to need the bathroom every couple of hours, rather than every twelve on the previous couple of days. According to the doctors this was an excellent sign that my body was finally starting to right itself and get rid of the accumulated fluid naturally. I can't tell you how relieved I was – the thought of a chest drain had been ever present in the back of my mind, and I was extremely grateful that it had been avoided.

However, once that worry disappeared it left more room for my other emotions about what was to happen the next day, Friday – two weeks since the embryo transfer. So far I'd had no bleeding and I was in the hospital with symptoms that often pointed to a successful treatment. The anticipation was deeply unsettling. Thursday evening came and went; I brushed my teeth, read my book, then switched off the light and tried to sleep. My chest had gradually felt a little better throughout the day, and the pressure had eased slightly so that it wasn't quite such a chore to breathe in. I lay there for a while but had to get up again to go to the bathroom. My eyes began to feel heavy, but my mind wouldn't let me sleep with its constant thoughts of what may happen the following morning.

Friday, 2nd September 2005
It was around 7.30 a.m. and the nurse had been to do my bloods. We had a chat afterwards and she said that I could do the pregnancy test, so she asked me how long it was since I'd been to the bathroom. As I knew my test was due that morning, and from experience that the concentration of the sample was all important, I'd made sure I hadn't gone for several hours.

I was so tired because I hadn't slept at all, having constantly tried to deal with my feelings regarding the test. It was the reason I was there after all and I'd been unable to get any peace from the thoughts whirling through my mind. Would it be positive, would it be negative, was having OHSS a sign that everything would be OK? The waiting was finally over; I hauled myself out of bed and into the bathroom. This was it – judgement day. I had no problem providing the sample and once back in bed I called the nurse. Now all I had to do was wait a few minutes and I would know.

Or so I thought. I waited; and waited; and waited.

What was going on? It should've only taken a couple of minutes, why hadn't anyone let me know? Half an hour went by; still nothing. Where the hell was the nurse, or the doctor, or anyone? Even the cleaner would do, as long as someone told me! I pressed my call button and a nurse finally arrived. I asked her what was happening and that I was waiting for the result of my pregnancy test. She looked a bit awkward and blank then just said that she didn't know and that she'd go and find out. For goodness sake, how difficult could it be? It was either positive or negative, why hadn't anyone been to tell me? Were they frightened to let me know if it was bad news? Had they lost the sample and I had to wait until the next day to do it again? I was going insane just not knowing anything. Another stressful half an hour later Mr Child finally arrived. At last, I thought, maybe I'd get my answer now.

He stood in front of me and said quite calmly that they'd done the test and that it was classed as a 'feint' positive with my hCG hormone level raised to twenty-five. However, it had only just scraped through and whilst it was good news, there was a need to be cautious as the hormone level should really have been a lot higher by this time. I didn't know what to think; I was pregnant but I wasn't pregnant. The cruel reality was that in theory the treatment had worked, but the signs weren't encouraging. Mr Child urged me to 'stay positive' and they'd do another test in a couple of days. He also spoke about letting me go home the next day depending on how well I did over the coming twenty-four hours. At least that was good news. I was fed up with being in the hospital, alone in my head and feeling like I was going through it all completely by myself. I realised that I needed family and friends around me to take my mind off things.

So, there I was in limbo. Neither certain nor uncertain of whether I was pregnant or not. I called James to let him know, but tempered the news with sobriety to make sure he didn't get too excited; the same went for my parents and my friend, Anna. Amazingly I managed to keep it together whilst I was on the phone. Somehow, something was telling me it wasn't going to be good news. The rational in me knew that trying to 'stay positive' wouldn't make a blind bit of difference and wouldn't alter the outcome. All that would do would give me false hope, so I succumbed to what my heart was telling me. I did find, however, that I couldn't shake this contradictory small light inside that said, "Yes, here I am, don't give up completely just yet." So I resolved to try and remain neutral for a couple more days – I'd have another test on Monday 5th when we'd know for definite. Until then I just had to get through the weekend.

The rest of Friday consisted of more of the same. A huge bouquet from Anna arrived, with a card that said "Congratulations" written on it. Whilst not wanting to sound ungrateful I actually felt sick when I saw it. It was a lovely thought but I found it inappropriate at that exact moment, and whilst I appreciated the effort and the fact that they were worried about me and wanted to make me feel better I just took one look at the flowers and felt really uneasy. It wasn't right; there wasn't anything to celebrate right now. I wished they'd have waited until after my second test.

The day went; the night came. I didn't sleep, but I did

cry. A lot. Again. On the one hand I felt as though I was the most unlucky, loneliest person in the world. On the other I felt guilty for feeling that way; there were people who were starving, or with incurable diseases, or had been in near fatal accidents who had to go through such a lot of physical, mental and emotional pain that I felt like a fraud. All I could do was try and justify in my mind that this was my experience, at this time in my life, and I didn't know any other way of handling it. If I felt this much angst, frustration and despair then it wasn't healthy to deny it and I just needed to allow myself to feel that way. The small light inside was still burning, if rather dimly, and as they say, "It isn't over 'til the fat lady sings", or whatever was politically correct to say these days.

Saturday, 3rd September 2005

Finally my chest was draining, although a bit slower than the doctors had hoped, so the decision was to keep me in until Monday, just to be on the safe side. My heart sank. It was only two more days but I was climbing the walls with boredom and the added worry about the 'sort of' positive pregnancy test meant that however hard I tried I just couldn't settle and think of anything else but that. My books didn't interest me, the magazines I had gave me a headache, there was nothing on TV except the horse racing and I couldn't access the internet, still, as no one had been to fix it. It was really sunny and warm and I was stuck inside. The food was, by now, less of a novelty and more of a necessity, and if I saw one more individually wrapped portion of cheese and crackers I'd throw it at the wall. Would someone *please* get me a Pot Noodle!

Sunday, 4th September 2005

Nonetheless, I managed to survive yet another day of 'nothing'. Why didn't hospitals arrange an on-site Starbucks for patients? I would've spent whole days in there sipping on chai tea lattes – at least you could get Wi-Fi internet access!

Sunday night came around and my thoughts turned to the fact that I'd be going home in the morning. Hopefully. My abdomen had quickly shrunk back to near normal proportions, although my legs were holding out, but as I still had to wear the lovely stockings it was nothing to worry about. I was happy about going home, but I knew that there'd also be another pregnancy test and I was deeply unsettled by it. I had a terrible feeling in the pit of my stomach that I tried to ignore. Despite everyone else's thoughts and their attempts at cajoling me into 'thinking positive', I knew what the outcome was going to be, no matter that a little shining something inside told me that I could be wrong. It was a real battle – a true case of head and heart contradicting each other, making my thoughts swing backwards and forwards, resulting in my mental state taking a real bashing and my emotions going from one extreme to the other. My last night in the hospital was not an easy one.

Monday, 5th September 2005

I was happy at the thought of going home to a comfortable bed and my own things around me. Funny how you miss such simple aspects of life and that they become so magnified when you're taken away from them, even for a short time.

A nurse came and took a blood sample – apparently it was the best way to get an accurate level of pregnancy hormone. James had arrived too and was busy getting my bag sorted when Mr Child knocked on the door to ask me to sign the release form, and to tell me to phone the fertility unit around 2 p.m. when they'd know the result of my test. I thanked him, checked the room to make sure I hadn't left anything behind, then we made our way out to the car park. It was weird walking out of the doors – I'd only been in the hospital for a week but as I'd been stuck inside all that time going outside again was so refreshing and the warm air felt wonderful.

We drove the short distance home – it was somewhat uncomfortable as I was still a little sore and bloated and my legs wouldn't function properly as they'd been strapped up in the stockings for so long. We hardly spoke during the journey; I think we were both just waiting for the next couple of hours to pass until we'd know for sure about the result. James was better at it than I was, or at least outwardly it looked to be that way. Once home he was able to get on with things in the office, while I just moped about and walked up and down pacing the floor of our apartment. He probably felt exactly the same as I did but he was better at compartmentalising, which allowed him to concentrate on other things.

I tried to eat some lunch but just couldn't face it. My stomach was all over the place and the built up expectation was awful. I lay down on the bed and closed my eyes for a while. My head hurt again from all the anxiety and my brain had been doing overtime going over and over everything constantly. I tried to zone out and focus on nothing but the thoughts just kept coming back. I put my headphones on and listened to Eros Ramazzotti, which helped a little then

I took a couple of paracetamol to try and dull the throbbing slightly. I glanced over at the clock; it was nearly 2 p.m.

I put my head round the door of the office and told James I was going to call the unit. I went into the living room, beautifully lit by the sun, where I sat on the edge of the sofa and dialled the number. It was answered almost immediately and I was put through to Mr Child. He started off by reconfirming that the result I'd had on Friday was a very low level of hCG hormone which was why they'd re-tested a sample. And then he just said it; unfortunately the new result had been zero, indicating a negative pregnancy test. He went on to say that I should expect to get some bleeding within a few days, pretty much like a normal period but it could be a bit heavier.

As soon as he'd said the word "unfortunately" the tears started to sting my eyes. By the time he'd got to the end of telling me about getting a bleed I was shaking. I needed to cry and only just managed to say, "OK". He said he was really sorry and that if there were any questions just to call straight back and someone would be able to help me. I couldn't talk any more; I was too choked inside and couldn't get my words out properly. I managed to garble that I had to go, put the phone down and let the tears take over. All the stress and emotional turmoil of the past seven months came out in floods. James had assumed the worst already and came over to hold me as I let out the emotion and pain. I sobbed uncontrollably and could hardly speak. Flying around in my head were the words, why? and, it's not fair, and all the other completely illogical thoughts that would torment me for months to come. My insides felt so empty; it was as if something had been taken away but without having had it in the first place. How hopeless and lonely I felt at that moment. I looked at James through swollen eyes and in between my tears kept saying, "I can't do it again. I'm really frightened."

I didn't know what to do with myself – my world had stopped once more. It was like floating whilst waiting for something to happen. James suggested I lie down and rest for a while, but I'd been doing that for a week in the damn hospital. I wouldn't be able to settle anyway – my emotions were all over the place. We chatted about things for a while, with me asking the unanswerable, "Why?" time and time again. After an hour or so I made myself a mug of tea, then, after having calmed down enough to have a semi-clear head decided to call Mr Child back to ask him a few questions.

The nurses were very understanding, and luckily they managed to put me through to him again. I asked why he thought I'd got pregnant and then had what was effectively a miscarriage. He explained that it was what they called a biochemical pregnancy – the hormone level is positive but very low and continues to decrease, meaning that whilst an embryo may have implanted it miscarries before being evident on an ultrasound scan. It was a very cruel 'successful' IVF cycle. According to Mr Child the fact that I did become pregnant was positive news in that it meant I could actually get pregnant from IVF again. Some consolation, I thought.

I asked him why I got OHSS, what I could have done any differently to change it, and whether having OHSS had been the cause of the miscarriage. He explained that given my health and background I was an unusual case in that I wasn't anywhere near what they would consider a risk.

I didn't fit any of the criteria and as such he wasn't able to give me any indication as to why – I was, "just unlucky". Nothing I had or hadn't done would've have prevented me from getting it, and it wasn't the cause of miscarrying. He went on to say that in fact, very often, when a woman experienced late onset symptoms it did point towards pregnancy, as the hormone levels had increased that much that OHSS could be one of the side effects of a successful IVF cycle. I considered this for a moment then asked him whether it may happen again. It was something that I was afraid of – I'd read that a couple of women had died from OHSS and it really frightened me to think that I could potentially be putting my life at risk; that there may be a reason why it happened to me particularly, and if that was the case was it worth doing all over again?

Unfortunately, Mr Child's answer was completely non-committal and neutral, as it had to be really. There was nothing anyone could do to guarantee I wouldn't get it again. All he could say was that the likelihood of getting it so severely in the first place was something like one per cent of all cycles, so the chances of it happening twice were even slimmer given that I still wasn't considered a high risk, even though my body had reacted in the way it did.

Mr Child recommended a follow-up appointment to discuss the cycle and decide what to do next. The dates he suggested were about two months away though – how on earth could I wait that long to discuss things? It was shocking – didn't they understand that people were in emotional pain and might need answers? The opportunity to talk it through with the 'professionals' would go some way to alleviating the feelings of desperation. Unfortunately, though, we just had to wait. Mr Child offered us his first free appointment which was 10th October – just over a month away.

I had no choice but to take it. Somehow I had to find a way of carrying on as normal for the next four weeks, but I knew I'd find it incredibly hard to focus on anything else. Mr Child also mentioned that there was a counselling service available and that if I felt I needed to discuss anything that was on my mind I could make an appointment to see someone at the hospital. At least it was better than nothing, but for the time being I decided to wait for our review appointment. James was happy to do this anyway – it hadn't affected him in the same way for obvious reasons, as he didn't have to deal with it on a physical level, and he hadn't got as caught up emotionally to the extent that I had. I put the phone down, surprisingly in a calmer frame of mind. It was only temporary though. I knew that I'd have moments of deep despair, but accepted that I simply had to deal with that when it happened.

Thursday, 8th September 2005

I was off work until the end of the week so my mum and dad arrived to spend the day with me. I still felt numb and didn't really want to do anything much, but I knew that was a sure-fire way to depression and feeling sorry for oneself, so I forced myself to go out for a while to have lunch and a coffee. It was only a short drive away so I suggested we went to Bicester Village Shopping Outlet as Oxford would be very busy. I needed a distraction other than just a walk somewhere.

We arrived late morning – it was surprisingly warm and sunny for September. Physically I felt a bit uncomfortable still, although not necessarily sore, and the bloating and swelling had completely disappeared. I think it was more to do with being sluggish and unfit – I hadn't been for a run or to the gym in weeks and my body felt heavy.

Lunchtime soon approached and we managed to find a table outside one of the cafés. I went inside to order with my dad whilst my mum stayed with the table, then we sat in the sun and ate our sandwiches. I watched people going by; mothers with prams, fathers with pushchairs, grandparents with toddlers. There suddenly seemed to be families everywhere I looked. I hadn't really noticed it before but it was polarised now and it made me feel empty. My dad started talking about my step-brother and his wife, and something their little boy had done at school recently. I felt my eyes smart and blinked a couple of times but it didn't work. I welled up and started to cry. I looked down into my lap to try and disguise the fact that I was upset, but nothing ever escaped my mum and she asked me what was wrong.

I said that I found it too upsetting talking about my brother and his kids. I apologised as it wasn't their fault, and my dad wasn't to know it would upset me. I didn't think it would either to be honest, but I obviously felt very raw still. My mum looked concerned and spoke gently that it would be alright. She nearly got upset for me too, bless her. My dad was a bit surprised that I'd had such a reaction to something so simple, but in my head I'd been replaying the 'what ifs' and 'that might never be me' scenarios. Once I'd let the emotion out though the temporary feelings started to subside. I knew they'd come and go like that, with nothing I could do to control the circumstances or the triggers. It was the 'so near but so far' truth that would haunt me for months to come – maybe I'd had my chance and it wasn't to be. Maybe this, and maybe that. I had to stop focusing on it, but I didn't know if I was capable.

Anyway, wobble over, we walked round the village for a while, but then went back home earlier than planned. There didn't seem to be any joy in just wandering aimlessly and I felt as if I was being a bit of burden to my mum and dad. Besides, I knew they had to get back home as they were both due at work the next day. A few hours later and after a light dinner, we said our goodbyes. I'd see them again in a couple of weeks' time.

Monday, 12th September 2005

I'd been thinking and thinking about our failed cycle ever since my parents left the previous Thursday. I tried not to let it occupy all my thoughts but, as usual, that was a very big ask. I really wanted to allow myself a few weeks until our appointment with Mr Child when not one thought or memory entered my head, but it seemed to be impossible. If anything I'd been thinking all the more which wasn't wise as I wasn't in possession of all the facts given we hadn't had our follow up meeting.

Over the previous four days I'd decided that the thing I needed to do to alleviate some of the feelings of being in limbo, was to take control of the situation as far as I could, so I contacted a very successful London clinic, the ARGC (Assisted Reproduction and Gynaecology Centre) in Harley Street, and asked them to send me their information so I could compare clinics. As soon as I'd done that it felt like things were moving again and I was doing something positive, rather than just waiting for bureaucracy to allow me to go to the next stage, whatever that may be.

When she called that night, I told my mum about the ARGC. I think she was just as frustrated as I was in that we had to wait for a process to occur with the John Radcliffe before we could move on. She was very encouraging when I told her, and said that she thought it was sensible to at least get information from other clinics. I also requested information from the ACU at UCH (Assisted Conception Unit at University College Hospital, now the CRGH; Centre for Reproductive and Genetic Health), in London, as I'd read that their success rates were also high.

It was during this telephone conversation that my mum mentioned my cousin and his wife again. Apparently their treatment had been successful and she was pregnant. Mum said she knew already the previous week but didn't feel she should say anything then as I'd been too upset when we went to Bicester. She'd been thinking in the meantime and had worried herself silly as to when to tell me.

The reason for that was that my grandma would be ninety in November and was having a party. I'd obviously be going, and so would my cousin and his wife, and she'd be at the point where her pregnancy would be obvious. My mum was really concerned about whether I'd be able to handle it, given what I'd gone through in the hospital, and the fact that people would be making a fuss, not knowing my history. She sounded relieved once she'd told me though. I said that yes, it would probably be difficult for me, but I had no plans to cancel and it would've been worse if no-one had told me beforehand. My brother, who lived in Germany, would also be there with his girlfriend, as would James obviously, and my mum and dad, so I'd be fine.

Inside though, I really wasn't looking forward to it as much as I should've been, but it was my grandma's party – it wasn't about me; it was about her, and I was determined to get through any tough moments somehow. We'd have had our follow-up meeting with Mr Child by then anyway, so we'd at least know about our options and have a plan.

So the days of September 2005 went by and I crossed them off the calendar one by one. It was just a countdown for me now until we met with Mr Child and decided on our next steps. I went to work as usual, came home and did some more work for James, then spent some time on the fertility support forum on the Fertility Friends website (www.fertilityfriends.co.uk), reading other people's questions and experiences to try and get an insight into reasons for my own. At work everything carried on as normal as no-one except my colleague, Ali, yet knew the real reason that I'd been in hospital for the week. She said several times that she thought I should tell my other colleagues, the directors that I worked for, but I still didn't feel comfortable with that. She assured me they'd completely understand, but nevertheless, it wasn't something I wanted to share at that point.

Monday, 10th October 2005
Our hospital appointment was in the morning so we drove the usual route and arrived in time to park the car in a side road round the corner. I didn't know how long we were going to be and it was always worth checking just to try and avoid the extortionate hospital car parking costs. Most of the road was reserved for residents' parking, but there was a small section that was available for anyone to use.

With fifteen minutes to spare we walked the short distance to the fertility unit. We hadn't been there long when we were called in to a consultation room, where a nurse confirmed who we were and that we were there to see Mr Child. It was a small, square room, decorated in blue with just a few soft chairs and a coffee table.

We sat down and prepared to wait, but to our surprise there was soon a knock on the door and Mr Child appeared. He asked how we'd been since the treatment a month ago, to which I said that it was obviously still upsetting and we felt as though we couldn't move on as we knew neither what the options were nor what the advice from the 'experts' was. He ran through the treatment plan and confirmed again that I didn't have any of the risk factors associated with ovarian hyperstimulation (under the age of thirty, very slim and/or underweight, polycystic ovarian syndrome, high hormone levels or high numbers of follicles and eggs collected). He said that the same could happen again and it was very difficult to quantify the risk. I mentioned that I had concerns about the long term complications of OHSS, but he told us that there were none known, as the condition was one that occurs then stops completely – an isolated condition if you like. If it did happen again all they'd be able to do would be admit me and manage it as before.

We'd already decided to try another cycle, even though the thought of what could happen made me feel sick inside, and full of worry and apprehension. I mentioned this to Mr Child who said that he completely understood how I felt, but he thought it was definitely worth trying another cycle, given that we were both otherwise healthy.

We finished our conversation on the understanding that I'd let the administrator know about our decision, and that I'd phone in when my next period appeared. I did wonder whether it was too early to try it again, given the huge amount of drugs involved, but after researching as much as I could there didn't seem to be any medical reason to wait. All that was required by the hospital was that I'd had at least one natural bleed before starting the process again, so with that due in early November I'd be in a position to start again for egg collection in December.

So, that was our decision. Despite the incredibly hard and most emotional few months we'd ever experienced we were going to put ourselves through it all over again. It would cost us financially too, but we really didn't feel we'd reached a stopping point. Finally there was a schedule of sorts and my head was free to move on a little. I felt somewhat calmer and better able to cope with the process of wondering and waiting, not to mention the further rounds of drugs that'd be required.

The administrator gave me a plan of booking in dates – a chart that listed the dates for the down regulation test and when to start the drug injections, depending on when my period was due. That was around 11th November, which unfortunately meant that I'd have to wait yet another month as the unit closed down for Christmas and my egg collection date would fall around that time. I was surprised to learn that the unit closed completely at Christmas and thought it absolutely ridiculous. I appreciated that people needed a break, especially at that time of year, but I thought at least they'd have some staff on. There was no point getting all worked up though. I needed to stay as calm and worry-free as possible to give myself a better chance of success second time around. It was only a month after all, and as my expected period date was very close to the cut-off, if it didn't arrive on time it could just push me into the next week anyway, making it irrelevant. I just had to hope that my November period was one of the longer cycles of thirty-three or thirty-four days.

Monday, 14th November 2005

And so it was – my period finally arrived meaning that I'd begin the down regulation drugs on 8th December, hopefully being ready for stimulation drugs on the 29th. My grandma's party had also been and gone, and I'd managed to get through it unscathed by throwing myself into the spirit of things, organising posters and getting celebratory newsletters printed.

Normally I was quite cheerful at this time of year and looked forward to Christmas but, naturally, my mind was on other things and I found myself wishing it would hurry up so we could get on with the treatment. I'd also been thinking about whether there was anything else I could do differently that would remove the connection in my mind to the last unsuccessful cycle and bad experience. My logic was that if I could do the cycle in a slightly different way, then it wouldn't be as easy to compare it with the first time, which would make me less inclined to focus on any similarities. It was a strange way to think I know, but it worked, and the thing that was different was that I decided to consult a western herbalist.

I'd read about how herbs could help many ailments, including the regulation of hormones. Of course, I did have a concern that it could interfere with the fertility drugs but after checking with the unit they said that as long as I wasn't taking anything during the stimulation phase then it wouldn't impact on the treatment in a negative way. Satisfied, I managed to find a local medicinal herbalist who'd been practicing for twelve years, often successfully treating women with recurrent miscarriage, and only prescribing western herbs, not Chinese. This was important to me as I wasn't comfortable in taking Chinese herbs, given that the eastern approach to taking them for medical reasons was completely different to that of western herbalism.

I arranged for an initial appointment that lasted about an hour or so where I was asked many questions about lifestyle and my previous history. Being a qualified herbalist, my practitioner tailored the contents of the tinctures specifically for me, given my state of health at the time. I decided to start with the herbs from just before my period was due, the 8th November, for just over two weeks. I was then prescribed a different mix from the 24th November to the 8th December, another again from the 8th to the 28th December, then a final mixture from 12th January for two weeks. The point of the mixtures was to regulate fluid balance, support the adrenal system, and to be calming and effective in reducing anxiety levels. It felt reassuring to me that at least I was trying to do something helpful and positive towards having a successful treatment cycle, and it definitely prevented me from focusing too much on the previous outcome, although admittedly, all the herbs tasted absolutely foul!

Chapter 5

Ding Dong, Round Two

Day one of our second IVF cycle finally arrived and on Thursday, 8th December 2005 I started to use the down-regulation nasal spray again. The next few days and weeks went by really slowly; I just wanted Christmas to hurry up and pass so I could start on the stimulation injections.

An impatient three weeks later I went for my hormone check – everything was at the right levels and I was given the go ahead to start the injections. I had no worries or concerns about injecting myself this time around – I was a pro by now, and didn't even think about it when I plunged the syringe into my stomach.

Wednesday, 4th January 2006

After seven days of injections I went to the hospital for my first scan to see how many follicles had developed. I'd been injecting 150 units of Gonal F per day, and my current E2 (estradiol hormone, connected to ovulation) level was 288. On the right ovary there were eight follicles measuring 12mm; 11mm; 9mm; 8mm; 8mm; 6mm; 6mm; and 5mm. The left ovary had five follicles measuring 12mm; 11mm; 6mm; 6mm; and 5mm. I was progressing slower than last time, but it was still early and there was approximately another week of stimulation to do.

Friday, 6th January 2006

This time my E2 was at 744 and the size of the follicles had increased, with an extra two on the left ovary. I was still on 150 Gonal F units per day and the decision was to carry on with this dose then rescan three days later.

Monday, 9th January 2006

With just a few days difference my E2 had reached 2,750 and another two follicles had appeared; the largest was now 21mm. It was time. I was given instructions to do the booster injection the following day, then after a day free of injections I was due to go in for egg retrieval on Thursday, 12th January 2006.

Wednesday, 11th January 2006

It was early evening and I'd started to get restless and apprehensive. My thoughts had turned to the 'what ifs' of the hyperstimulation happening again. I tried to ignore them but they was always there, niggling away. So far I'd managed to deal with it quite well and had surprised myself by how composed I was. But now it was crunch time once more and I was faced with the two week wait yet again, knowing that not only would I be thinking about whether the treatment had worked, but also whether I'd get ill from it. In the end I just had to get on with it. There was nothing I could do now – it had been my choice to do another cycle and I knew it was a risk, probably even more so than the first, probably not, so I just had to take the responsibility for my choice. After mulling it over for a while I became quite cavalier about it, which I think helped me to be more rational and allowed me to stop indulging myself in the negative possibilities.

So with that worry dealt with my thoughts turned to the actual process of the egg collection. I couldn't remember it from the first time, so this helped for the second time in that I knew it wasn't going to hurt, but even if it did I wouldn't recall it anyway due to the sedation. With a calm mind I went to bed at around 9 p.m. We had to be up fairly early as the collection was scheduled for 9.45 a.m., and I knew I'd need all the energy I could muster to get through the coming days.

Thursday, January 12th 2006

It was around 9.30 a.m. and as I waited to go into the collection room once more I couldn't help but wonder how many eggs there'd be this time. It was a daft thing to be concerned about really as the quantity of eggs collected had absolutely no bearing on the quality, or potential success. There could be twenty-five and none of them would be of a high enough standard, or there could be three or four of such good quality that there'd be a couple left over to freeze.

We waited a bit longer then a nurse called our names and checked her notes to make sure we matched their records. James was called first to do his 'thing', then a few minutes later I was back in the chair in the same room as before, with the anaesthetist chatting away and beginning to administer the sedation. My stomach rumbled as she did so; I was absolutely starving as I wasn't allowed to eat anything until after the procedure. Images of bacon sandwiches floated around my head, which was a bit bizarre as I never ate them.

It suddenly dawned on me that I was about to put

myself through the same stomach churning, unsettling and worrying two weeks yet again. I was still contemplating this when I felt my eyes become heavy, then everything went completely blank until I came round a short while later in the recovery area.

The first thing I said when I opened my eyes was, "How many did we get this time?" My mum, who was sat in the chair next to the bed, told me that they'd collected nine. I looked from her to James and back again, then waited for the inevitable pang of disappointment, as I just said, "Oh." It was only three less than last time, but still, given that there'd been no embryos to freeze then my logic said that the more eggs collected the better, irrational as that was and completely contradictory to what I'd thought only a few hours ago. Instead of being happy with the achievement of nine, all my head seemed to hear was that there were three less. I knew I sounded ungrateful so I tried not to let it show that it bothered me. After a lot of thought I managed to convince myself that maybe the eggs would be of better quality, meaning potentially better quality embryos. There would've been no point in asking the nurse what her thoughts were as she'd only have been non-committal, so I put it to the back of my mind realising that worrying about something I couldn't change was a complete waste of time.

Before I could be released a nurse checked to see if I was able to walk without feeling woozy, then, armed with the usual hormonal suppositories and strict instructions to rest I was allowed to go home. Given the OHSS of the first cycle I was also warned to make sure I notified the hospital straight away if I started to feel out of breath and overly bloated. They had no worries on that score though, as I knew it would be constantly on my mind for the whole of the next two weeks.

Friday, 13th January 2006
On waking I immediately checked to see how much bloating and soreness I had, but surprisingly it was minimal and I actually felt OK. After a late breakfast and feeling refreshed following a shower, the phone rang – it was a nurse at the hospital calling to say that six of the eggs had fertilised and that the transfer was definitely booked in for the next day, Saturday, 14th January. We actually had one more successfully fertilised egg than last time, which was very encouraging. I found that I was a lot calmer than before too – the unexpected had become the familiar.

The rest of the day passed without incident. My mum left late morning to go home as she had to be at work the next day. After she left I spent more time internet researching to try and find about how other people had spent the dreaded 'two week wait'. I'd already done this once before of course, during the first cycle, but I thought there could be some more information out there that I missed the first time around. It must've been several hours later that my head started to hurt with reading the screen so intensely, so I watched some rubbish TV instead. What I really wanted to do was go out for some fresh air, but as it was a cold and windy January day, and I was unable to drive myself anywhere I didn't have any choice but to stay put. On went the kettle yet again and I settled down with my hot water bottle, a cup of tea and a book. A couple of hours later James got back from work, producing dinner courtesy of Marks and Spencer, thankfully, as I really didn't feel like cooking anything. After an early meal I put my headphones on and listened to Eros Ramazzotti, losing myself in the music in an attempt to still my mind. It worked, and an hour later, after a warm bath and still in a rare moment of serenity, I went to bed.

Saturday, January 14th 2006

Embryo transfer was scheduled for 10 a.m., but I'd planned to be there much earlier as I had an acupuncture session immediately beforehand. Anna came with me this time around, and as we sat in the car on the way to the hospital she asked me how I felt. Apprehensive and nauseous was probably the best way to describe it. After the ease of egg collection my insides had decided to give me a hard time – it was probably the adrenalin giving me the shakes.

Weekend traffic was definitely easier to navigate and we soon arrived at the hospital. My acupuncturist was already waiting, and once we'd done the security check I assumed we'd be given a room in which to do the acupuncture. However, we were asked to sit in the reception area with no explanation other than that a nurse wouldn't be too long. So we sat for ten minutes, then another ten minutes, then I started to get anxious. Keeping people waiting when they were having treatment, without a reason, really wasn't acceptable. My acupuncturist wondered what on earth was going on, as she needed at least forty-five minutes to complete the session.

Finally a nurse appeared and said that they were running a bit late due to a complicated egg collection, but she'd found a room available for us to use for the acupuncture. Relieved, we made ourselves comfortable in one of the scanning rooms, where there was a bed and a couple of chairs. It was important during the acupuncture session that I tried to relax to enable it to work properly, but I was already a bit agitated by the delay. Surely the staff should've known how unnerving it'd be, shouldn't they? Maybe it was just me being a bit too sensitive, but then to me it was a sensitive time and it would've been nice to have had an explanation a bit earlier on. Still, there was no point in focusing on that now – I had to get in the right frame of mind.

After I'd made myself comfortable on the bed the practitioner began to insert the needles. Every time she placed a new one I had to mention when I felt the familiar dragging sensation, so that she knew it was in exactly the right position. Once they were all inserted she left Anna and me alone whilst the needles worked their 'magic'. We chatted for a bit, mostly about how her work was going and what she and her husband had planned for the rest of the weekend. I tried to empty my thoughts of anything negative although it was pretty difficult – it wasn't exactly the optimum environment in which to switch off.

Twenty minutes or so later the acupuncturist came back in and removed the needles. I told the receptionist that I was ready and she said they'd just be a few more minutes. No sooner had we picked up a magazine than the lead nurse arrived to call us through.

It was the same room that I was used to and as I tried to make myself comfortable on the bed, Anna pulled up a nearby spare chair. The nurse began by explaining that there were two embryos to transfer, and that another one was of good enough quality to freeze for a later cycle if necessary. I had to decide before I left the hospital if I wanted to do that, as it had to be frozen as soon as possible. I was really pleased that we had one to freeze; we hadn't been that lucky in the previous cycle. I decided there and then that we'd keep it in storage, whatever the extra cost. I was sure that this cycle was going to work but you never knew so I wanted to make sure we had an alternative just in case.

The nurse also told me that it wasn't a doctor who'd be doing the transfer this time as it was the weekend, but a nurse, who was apparently very experienced. I was quite surprised and not too pleased about that. It was, after all, a very tricky procedure and I really wanted a doctor to do it, but I didn't have any choice. It had to be done now and no-one else was available. I didn't understand why they didn't have a rule of only doctors to do collections and transfers; it was as if it really didn't matter. Well, it did to me, and I was very annoyed. There was nothing I could do though, and I realised that there was no point in making it an even bigger issue – that would have just wound me up and made me stressed. I reminded myself how often they did these procedures and that it really would be alright.

I was gazing at the ceiling when the nurse told me she was about to insert the catheter. As before, there was a small screen next to the bed so it was possible to see when the embryos were transferred. Not that I could see much as it was all a blur – you had to be a scan specialist to be able to tell which bit was which on the ultrasound. Suddenly I felt a very uncomfortable dragging and heavy feeling inside which I didn't experience during the first transfer. I told the nurse that it hurt a little and was very uncomfortable at which point she said that they were having difficulty inserting the catheter.

Apparently there was a slight kink at the entrance to my uterus and the catheter wouldn't go round it properly. I thought that was incredibly odd – there hadn't been a problem during the first transfer procedure. After a change of catheter type the nurse tried again, and luckily this time it was successful. I could see on the screen that she adjusted it in and out a bit, then finally she said that the embryos were right at the end of the catheter, then that they'd been released. She called to a colleague to check that the catheter was empty, who confirmed that it was, and that was it. My second embryo transfer was done.

I hadn't noticed anything happen at all on the ultrasound screen, and neither had Anna. During the first embryo transfer I could clearly see two small dots but this time I saw nothing. I was quickly rushed up and out of the chair and shown back to the room where I was having the acupuncture treatment post-transfer. It all happened in a bit of a blur and I could feel myself getting upset. I got the impression that no-one was really bothered or cared about the feelings of patients – it was as though patient care had been forgotten about and it made me feel like I was back on that production line again.

I thought about it for a while as the acupuncturist inserted the needles; this time in slightly different places. Once she'd finished she left Anna and me alone again but I didn't feel like chatting this time. I hoped that Anna wasn't bored to tears as she'd just been hanging around really, and I felt a bit awkward as if I was wasting her time. Not that she gave me that impression; it was probably just me being hyper sensitive by the whole experience. My head was all over the place and I felt unsettled. I just wished that the procedure had gone more smoothly and I'd been treated as if I was an individual with real emotions and feelings. The staff did this for a living so they probably just saw it as a process, and I was one of many.

The practitioner returned to see how I was getting on and to check that none of the needles had fallen out. As she was doing so we heard a knock at the door and a doctor appeared. With a serious and straight face she asked us if we thought we'd be much longer as they wanted to close. I couldn't believe it and was stunned into silence – one minute we were told they were running late, the next they had the cheek to ask us to hurry up as they wanted to get off home!

Eventually we left the hospital and Anna dropped me back at our apartment. I kept replaying everything in my mind. Not that I wanted to dwell on it but I just couldn't help analysing every bit of the procedure. I wished my brain would forget and let me have some peace for a change, rather than giving me constant pressure in my head from all the thinking. The only respite came when I slept, which I did plenty of that afternoon. Unfortunately I was woken up by some quite sharp cramping inside, although I didn't panic. It was to be expected really, even though I didn't experience any after the first transfer. It was always a comparison with the first time – everything I did or didn't do I compared to how it was 'the first time'. It was very frustrating.

Monday, 16th January 2006

Nothing. No cramps; no pain; no bloating. I was off work for the whole two weeks this time as I didn't want to take any chances. On the other hand, maybe resting so much wasn't a good idea – perhaps I needed to move a bit more to get the blood flowing round my system. I couldn't decide which to do. Last time I didn't really rest, but then I didn't tire myself out either. In the end I walked round the apartment, backwards and forwards from one room to the next; it wasn't as if I could go outside anyway as it was too cold. Bored of that after ten minutes, I decided to log on to the Fertility Friends support website to see who was doing what and when.

I scanned the forum for any new questions or posts. I spotted two BFPs (big fat positive) from a couple of posters I'd corresponded with previously, so sent congratulations. I still felt a bit upset and angry about Saturday's shenanigans so I wrote a post about the experience and how the hospital staff had upset me by trying to rush me out of the door that day. Typing it out and telling someone else about it – someone who'd been through the same thing – helped me to get it out of my head. There were a couple of reassuring responses too – someone else also had a similar experience and got a positive pregnancy test so it did placate me somewhat. I spent the next hour or so reading posts, followed by yet another internet search on OHSS; how to avoid it, how risky it is etc. Not that it did me any good but I thought that maybe there was some information I hadn't found yet – again. I've mentioned that once already I think – you can see how IVF completely takes over your life.

Tuesday, 24th January 2006

It was day eleven of fourteen and I'd had an uneventful past ten days. I'd been watching the news on Sky when I decided to make some tea. I got up to go to the kitchen but went to the bathroom first, and it was then that I noticed a pink discharge. It wasn't a bleed as such but I knew that it definitely shouldn't have been there. I forgot about the tea and switched on my laptop so I could check the internet for 'discharge after embryo transfer'. It was all very confusing – it could be the start of my period or it could be implantation bleeding which would mean a successful transfer – so that wasn't much use then. I suppose I was looking for reassurance and confirmation, but somehow I just knew it was over. Again, gut feeling told me that it wasn't going to happen and the transfer had failed.

I rang my mum and told her that I knew it hadn't worked. She tried to say that it wasn't necessarily the case and that we wouldn't know until a few days' time when I could do the pregnancy test. She told me to stay positive, it could still be alright, but I knew in my heart that it wasn't. I already suspected it wouldn't work straight after they did the transfer. The whole thing just didn't go right and I'd been left with the awful feeling of it having been a wasted cycle. Some would say that I was negative about it, but it wasn't about that – it was about being realistic. I'd considered the cycle in a logical way, weighing up the facts of what happened, and it just didn't equate to success. There probably wasn't even any link to emotional wellbeing at the time of and just after embryo transfer; who's to say whether a state of mind could affect implantation or not? We know that it can affect many health problems, but surely that was over time, not just over a couple of hours. In my opinion, all the 'positive thinking' in the world wouldn't make a blind bit of difference to something that was purely biological.

Looking for something to blame though, I couldn't help but focus on the fact that my mental state had suffered from the huge swings of emotions involved in the entire process right from the beginning, and that if my character had been one of a more laid-back disposition the whole thing may have turned out so differently. There was absolutely no point in beating myself up about that though; there was nothing I could do to change it or my character. My only available option was to try and cope with it; besides, there were still four more days to go until we'd know for sure.

Saturday, 28th January 2006
The fat lady sang.

Chapter 6

Time for a Change

The failure of cycle number two came as no surprise really. As I mentioned, my gut feeling was that it had been a waste of time since the day of embryo transfer. Not that I could possibly ever know why it didn't work, but it seemed that fate had decided it wasn't to be. Strangely, although obviously upset, I felt more able to deal with it than the first time, probably because of the OHSS circumstances, but also I think because I'd already allowed myself to accept it over the previous two weeks whilst waiting to take the pregnancy test. Of course it was still completely heart-breaking and the worry in my head had turned to the 'what if it doesn't happen, ever' scenario. I was concerned about finances for one thing, and for another I didn't want to keep risking my health over and over again, not just physically but mentally and emotionally too. I was resilient, but I knew I'd have a breaking point somewhere and I didn't know when that would be; James and I had some hard thinking to do before we planned our next step.

Like the first time, I wanted to make absolutely sure we made the right decision before going for another cycle. Not that I would've considered stopping just yet – I wasn't ready to do that so I knew there'd be another attempt, but I was no longer convinced that the fertility unit in Oxford was the right place for us. There was also the frozen embryo we could use, although if we did we'd definitely be tied to having the cycle in Oxford. It would be possible to transfer the embryo to another hospital but I'd never be able to forgive myself if something went wrong and we lost it completely. We had to chat to Mr Child in an attempt to decide what to do, so I phoned the fertility unit on the Saturday morning of the failed cycle and asked if I could sort out a date for our follow-up appointment. We were lucky – there was a spare slot in his diary for 13th February 2006. That was only a couple of weeks away, and it would give us some time to think about our options.

I went back to work straight away the following week. It was a good distraction for me as it meant I was busy and didn't have the time to dwell on things. At least not in the mornings anyway – in the afternoons, if I wasn't doing some admin work, I found myself researching on the internet. It was during one of these afternoons that I investigated some other clinics, in addition to those London ones I'd already received information about. I looked at the various success rates, where they were in the country, whether it would be possible to travel to somewhere else, and what other couples had experienced in terms of the service and professionalism of the staff etc. I seriously looked at a clinic near Cambridge; I think it was Bourn Hall, and called them to ask about their procedures and how they monitored their patients. I spoke to a nurse and asked them to post their literature, then dug out the information on the London clinics and began to read through it again. I also looked at their websites – the ARGC (Assisted Reproduction and Gynaecology Centre) was quite impressive, with the highest success rate in the country. I thought it might be an idea to chat to someone to find out a bit more, so I dialled the number and waited for someone to answer. I was disappointed when no-one did though, and I had to leave an answerphone message – hmmm. I told myself not to be judgmental when I hadn't even spoken to anyone yet and that it was probably just because they were so busy, although admittedly I didn't think it was a good omen. I berated myself again then decided it wouldn't do any harm in making an appointment for a consultation.

The other London clinic's website caught my eye too – it gave the impression of being really friendly, but for some reason I assumed that it would be way too expensive and just as impractical as the ARGC location-wise. It was the Assisted Conception Unit at the University College Hospital. I waited for the Cambridge clinic to send me their information pack then, once it arrived a few days later, I settled down one evening to compare the three that I'd selected. James was happy to let me make the decision in terms of where we had the next treatment, which may seem strange, but his logic was that I was the one going through the physical aspect of treatment so it should be up to me to decide where I wanted that to happen. Besides, he knew how methodical and diligent I was and he had faith that my decision would be the right one. After several hours of lists and note-taking, I'd at least come to the conclusion that Bourn Hall in Cambridge was no longer in the running. Partly because it didn't 'feel' like the right one, and partly because I'd also been researching a different type of embryo transfer, and they wouldn't necessarily offer it given our history.

To explain, whilst trying to find out why both our treatments had failed, I repeatedly came across a type of embryo transfer that statistically had a better chance of success; blastocyst. This is an embryo that has had the chance to develop for longer than the usual two to three days before being transferred back into the uterus. It's cultured in the laboratory for a period of between five and six days, which allows the embryologist to select the strongest of multiple embryos to transfer. It's not recommended for all patients though, as not all embryos are strong enough to reach that point and stop developing after day two or three, increasing the risk of not having any embryos to transfer. It's often recommended for patients with many good quality eggs but previous failed IVF treatments, as the chances of success are much higher if the five or six day target is reached.

When I first read about it it sounded perfect and I was convinced I'd found the solution. I researched and researched and researched, and the more I discovered the more it appeared to be the obvious answer for us. Suddenly a small ray of hope appeared. Obviously I was no medical expert, but I was completely sure that it could work. With only a week until our follow-up appointment with Mr Child, my mood lifted. I couldn't wait for us to discuss it with him as I felt sure he'd agree that it was the best thing to do.

Monday, 13th February 2006

Our appointment wasn't until 3 p.m. but I was on edge all morning. We knew the drill as we'd been there before, but this time it was different. I think in my heart I'd already made my mind up not to have another cycle with the Oxford clinic, but I wanted this appointment still as I needed some kind of sign that it was the right decision. I'm not sure what I was looking for exactly but I knew something would happen or be said during conversation that would be the confirmation I was looking for. Gut feeling again I suppose.

Anyhow, we made our way to the hospital after a late lunch, spent about half an hour looking for a parking space as the side road was occupied, and arrived in reception with about ten minutes to spare. I got déjà vu big time – Radio 2 playing, flowers in vases, patients waiting. It was a bit daft really as of course it would be the same as before, except this time I didn't look at the other couples and wonder what they were going through – I already knew. I did notice how calm they appeared though; not that I expected them all to be in floods of tears and looking as miserable as a wet weekend. Maybe they were all so blank because they were in their own world, just as I was.

I carried on reading my magazine while the nurses came and went calling names and checking that they were speaking to the right people, then after five minutes or so it was our turn once again. The nurse showed us to a small consulting room off the main corridor in which were three chairs and a small table, and said that Mr Child wouldn't be long.

We sat down and looked at each other with a sigh of, "hey-ho, here we are again then". James had brought a pen and a pad with him and scribbled notes and equations about work on it. Clouds had gathered outside and it had turned grey; rain started to run down the window pane. I sighed. I felt tired, deflated, and terribly sad – I think it was the thought of having to go through the whole draining chaos of it once more. I just wanted to get the consultation over with to satisfy my mind.

My thoughts were interrupted by a knock on the door and Mr Child appeared. He shook our hands and welcomed us, albeit under unfortunate circumstances yet again. He sat down opposite James and me and asked how I felt. I said that I was disheartened and disappointed that the second cycle hadn't worked, that I was confused as to why, and that maybe there could be an underlying reason. He mentioned that on average it took two or three cycles to be successful and that it was by no means unusual. He went on to say that my physiology looked perfectly fine so it did just seem to be a matter of having been unlucky, as the embryos that were transferred on the second cycle were of high quality. I paused for a moment then asked him whether we could try a blastocyst transfer cycle, to which he looked slightly surprised. I didn't know why though, unless he just wasn't used to patients being so straightforward, asking questions about medical procedures. Perhaps he thought we shouldn't interfere in the 'science' of it all and just do what we were told. His initial reaction confirmed everything to me – it was the sign I needed, and I was now one hundred per cent sure that our third and final cycle would be with a different clinic.

I mentioned there and then that we'd researched other clinics and had decided that we needed to move on from Oxford, given our history of failed cycles. I said that I wasn't comfortable having what would be our last attempt at the John Radcliffe, and that psychologically I wanted the freshness of a new environment. Mr Child appeared to understand and didn't try to change our minds. The conversation came to an end and Mr Child said goodbye and good luck, then went off to arrange for a nurse to let us have some forms to sign, and to sort out copies of our previous blood tests and history so we could let our new clinic have some background information. We only waited a couple of minutes when the nurse appeared, armed with the relevant items – we'd never experienced such a prompt service before.

As she sat down and we signed the release forms, she asked us which clinic we'd chosen for our last treatment. When I mentioned it was in London she immediately asked if it was the ARGC. She advised us to make sure we knew what we were doing as they sometimes suggested extra tests that not many other clinics offered and that we could end up not being successful anyway. I was rather taken aback at her comments, and just mentioned that we'd considered several options and hadn't made our final decision yet. She made me feel very uncomfortable – sort of guilty for wanting to try another clinic and I just wanted to get out of the door and go home. I wanted to forget about the negative experiences we'd had at the John Radcliffe and focus on the potential of our last attempt somewhere else, somewhere positive, somewhere new.

Thursday, 16th February 2006

We received our appointment by post for the ARGC in Harley Street. It was arranged for the beginning of May; quite a way off, but given their excellent reputation not as far as I'd expected. I called to confirm, at which point I was told that I'd have to have some blood tests done on the day and it would be around £350. I asked if it was really necessary given that we'd already had all the relevant blood tests because of our previous attempts, but unfortunately they did have to be done again. As the original bloods had been tested about a year earlier they weren't considered recent enough – things could have changed during that time and we definitely needed to have them refreshed. The nurse did advise us that we could try and get them done locally on the NHS via our GP. Some people were able to do that apparently, but it did depend on whether the GP was happy to authorise it, given that the treatment itself was private. It was worth asking though, so I made a note to request an appointment at the local doctors' surgery in the meantime. We knew that private treatment would cost us more but given we'd already spent around £8,000 on the two previous ICSI attempts, £350 just for pathology before we'd even started was rather unexpected.

I made myself a cup of tea then switched on my laptop and logged on to the ARGC section of the Fertility Friends website. I started to read the posts from other women who'd undergone treatment there, and after reading a few comments I noticed that there was a common thread specific to that particular clinic – something called IVIG (intravenous immunoglobulin).

Apparently, one of the reasons that the ARGC clinic's results were so high could be that they recommended this therapy for women who'd had previous attempts at fertility treatment without success. I read on a bit to see if anyone mentioned what was involved in the treatment, after which a small spark of doubt in the back of my mind wouldn't go away. Given our history of two failed cycles, the first step after a consultation could be an immune blood screening profile, involving a series of vials of my blood being sent to the USA to be analysed for something called NK cells. For some women who suffered from miscarriages or unsuccessful IVF treatments, it could be because cells in their blood reject an embryo when it implants. If the analysed blood samples showed an increased level of these NK cells, then the ARGC may recommend IVIG treatment prior to the traditional treatment of IVF/ICSI. It involved administering antibodies extracted from the blood plasma of many different donors, and is given by intravenous drip[ii]. Several sessions would be required – during stimulation phase and then again a couple of weeks after implantation if the pregnancy test result was positive.

I sat for a while and considered all this extra information regarding IVIG therapy. There looked to be quite a lot of women who'd been through it and, becoming pregnant, thought it was the most fantastic thing ever, and that it was the reason why they finally had a successful cycle. Whether IVIG really was the reason would never be known – the fact that they'd had a successful cycle was enough to convince them that it had made the difference, and if I was put in the same position I'd probably think the same. I read on a bit more, reviewing some other posts. It struck me as being an obvious choice, so why then, did I still feel uneasy? As usual I'd got way ahead of myself – it might not even be recommended for us, although I did believe that if we went for our consultation it'd be exactly what would be suggested.

It wasn't only that though – a very small, what some people would call quite trivial, doubt also bothered me. As I'd read through the posts in the forum about the experiences and questions of other women at the ARGC, it became clear that the clinic was very much in demand. So in demand, in fact, that it often seemed, when patients had gone for treatment, there wasn't any room left in the waiting area. Being honest with myself, how would I handle that situation? If I was due to go in for egg collection or embryo transfer and found myself one of many, jostling for space whilst nurses rushed about with many different patients I'd be in a right panic. No way would I be able to deal with that, and I knew I'd get very stressed.

I tried to get it in perspective, weighing up the pros of having treatment at one of the best clinics in the UK, with the fact that I felt uneasy about both IVIG therapy and maybe feeling like I was 'just a number'. I needed some other points of view, so I posted a message on the forum explaining my fears. One poster said she'd recently transferred to the ARGC and had her blood sent to Chicago for analysis – all seventeen vials full. Several other responses mentioned that IVIG hadn't even been mentioned at their consultations, and I got the impression that most women were happy and comfortable with the clinic. Maybe I was the crazy one then! I logged out of the site to try and forget about it for a while – a good night's sleep would give me a clearer head.

Friday, 17th February 2006

I went to work as usual and busied myself doing routine tasks, all the time waiting for one o'clock to come around so I could go home. I decided to stop by the gym on the way – I hadn't been for ages and always felt better after a run and a session on the cross-trainer. The good thing about going in the middle of the day was that you missed both the lunchtime and evening rush for equipment. I'd often had the pool all to myself for the whole time; until I decided not to swim any more since I started thinking about the chlorine in the water and whether it could affect my health. Sometimes I wish I didn't think so much – it would make things a little bit easier. That's what happens when you're left to your own devices I suppose; too much time to ponder.

I finally got home at about 3 p.m. I'd been considering my thoughts about the ARGC from the day before and decided to post another question on the Fertility Friends forum. Several other queries had come up and I wanted to see what other people thought and whether they'd had any experience with these particular issues. One of the things I asked about was the potential effect of immune testing and any subsequent therapy on my ability to gain life and/ or health insurance in the future. For instance, whether the fact of just being tested automatically ruled out certain elements of a life insurance policy. Whilst not currently having one, it was something we'd been considering and although it may not be a deciding factor it would still contribute to our decision as to whether or not to proceed, if we were indeed advised to have immune testing and IVIG. Having to potentially take drugs in addition to the IVF ones still really bothered me too, never mind the thought of a blood transfusion for a reason that wasn't life-threatening. It just didn't sit right with me.

Within half an hour of posting I'd had a couple of responses to my question. One of the ladies was in a similar situation, but with only one failed ICSI treatment. She said that as she'd already had a negative cycle, the doctor would consider immune testing. It wasn't suggested that she do it but she'd decided to anyway to find out if there were any issues. I thought about this for a moment and tried to apply it to our situation. In my heart I knew there weren't any problems relating to my chemistry or biology. Some would probably say that I was fooling myself by thinking it wasn't 'my' issue if I didn't find out for sure through testing, but to me that argument wasn't good enough given my strong feelings.

A couple of minutes later another response appeared. This time it was from someone who had similar thoughts to me. As well as having been told by a different clinic that in their opinion it was pure bad luck that a negative cycle had happened, the extra timescale involved in testing seemed to be a factor in her consideration. Like me, she had normal levels of everything that had already been tested for by way of standard blood tests e.g. hormone levels etc., and something was telling her not to go for immune testing/IVIG either. Another posting, and this time the ARGC advised that as the lady concerned had two negative attempts behind her, it might be a good idea to have immune testing done.

So now I had a fair mix of thoughts and opinions, which made me feel slightly better that I wasn't alone in my worries, although my head started to hurt again – too much information to mull over. With a couple of months before the ARGC could see us, I decided to use the time productively by arranging for my standard repeat blood tests through my GP and trying to relax ready for our last attempt.

Friday, 24th March 2006

It was eleven o'clock in the morning and I was sat in a very busy waiting room. I had an appointment with the nurse at my local surgery to have a blood test to check for the level of progesterone. This is the hormone that prepares the body for an embryo and supports implantation, and it has to be within a certain range to ensure the environment in the uterus is optimal. I'd had to use a kit to pinpoint exactly when ovulation had occurred so I could have the test done on the right day.

I'd also had another series of blood tests a few weeks earlier to check for the hormones estradiol, LH, FSH and prolactin, and a full blood count. My results all came back completely normal with a progesterone level of fifty-four and full blood count within expected ranges. In fact, I decided to research blood count ranges on the internet, so I could see for myself what was normal and what was not etc., and the count for lymphocytes, which relates to immunity and the NK cells, amongst others, was completely within the usual range. My mind started whirring again. If those levels were normal surely then our problem was not one of immunity? It was all I needed to know to confirm that IVIG therapy wasn't for us, regardless of whether my conclusion was medically accurate or not; to me it was enough of a reason. I was satisfied with my decision and whilst we still had to deal with another cycle of fertility treatment, the thick fog had turned into a thin mist.

Saturday, 25th March 2006

A letter arrived from the other London clinic, UCH, confirming an appointment for the afternoon of 10th April

2006, when we were booked in to see Mr Paul Serhal. I decided to google his name and what I found was very encouraging. Given how I always liked to see the 'top' man or woman for absolutely anything, even if having my hair cut, the fact that Mr Serhal founded the unit at UCH and was considered one of the best experts in the fertility field, I thought being referred to him straight away was the best possible chance we were going to get to finally be successful. This was before we'd even met him. Intuition told me that UCH was for us, and the ARGC wasn't. However, I still didn't feel ready to make the final decision until I'd been to the appointments. I wasn't going to decide something that would affect the rest of our lives without considering all the options. I was convinced there would come a time, very shortly, when I would know exactly what to do for the best – I wasn't sure when that time would be but I knew that I'd recognise the moment and be one hundred per cent sure. All I had to do was wait a little while longer and the right decision would find me.

Chapter 7

The Right Choice

Monday, 10th April 2006

Our appointment with UCH had finally arrived and I'd arranged to travel down to London by train to meet James at his office before going to the clinic. We didn't have to be there until 3.30 p.m. but I decided to go quite a bit earlier so I could relax and have some lunch on my own beforehand. I was hyped up and couldn't figure out why – it was only an appointment, although it probably had something to do with the fact that this would be our last chance and I was pinning all my hopes on UCH being perfect. Setting myself up to potentially be disappointed didn't even calculate; I so hoped that everything was going to be right, feel right, look right – including a comfortable environment and great staff with really positive attitudes. I just knew that I'd know, if you see what I mean.

I finished work early so I could take a late morning train and sat gazing out of the window – it would become something of a ritual over the next couple of months. It was strangely soothing to just sit there with a clear head, being neither here nor there, preparing myself for another appointment.

The train arrived on time and after ordering a chai tea latte to go at Starbucks I made my way to Mayfair to meet James. I decided to walk from Paddington – it only took half an hour anyway, and I preferred it to the bus or the underground. When I arrived at his office building my nervousness returned, although it was mixed with a sense of optimism. I was impatient to get to the clinic and our appointment so we immediately set off to Green Park to take the underground to Kings Cross station.

The clinic was on Grey's Inn Road and only a five minute walk away from the railway station. We arrived at the main front doors and made our way up the steps, slightly concerned that the sign at the front said Eastman Dental Clinic, and nothing about an IVF unit. There were no signs in the lobby that said anything relating to the fertility unit either, so we wandered aimlessly for about five minutes thinking we must have missed the entrance further down the road. We finally asked someone (James had been insistent on not asking for directions, of course) and after being directed through a couple of double doors and down several corridors with pictures of teeth on the walls, we arrived at what looked like a small reception area.

It was screened off from the corridor by a wall with privacy glass windows across the top half, and as I popped my head round the side and saw posters and photos of babies, I realised we were in the right place. I smiled at the receptionist and said we were there to see Mr Serhal. Our names were ticked off in the appointment book then we were asked to sit down and wait. One thing that struck me whilst we were waiting was the quietness of the place. People were repeatedly called for scans or checks, or to settle their bills, and it came across as being very organised and serene. Even though the hospital was in the middle of

London and it was a large building, it felt very personal. Being built in the 1930s, it had thick walls, old radiators and huge high windows. Usually I preferred more modern buildings but for the purpose of our treatment, this one felt comforting.

After a few minutes we were called into a consulting room where a nurse explained that James would have to provide a sample, which would be analysed there and then so that we'd know the results. A plan would then be suggested directly after our consultation with Mr Serhal.

I was astounded; it took a whole week last time as the results had to be sent back via our GP. This time we had to pay £95 for the sample test and £180 for the consultation, but the difference between private and NHS was already evident.

As James disappeared down the corridor I sat in the reception area to wait again. I was nervous at the thought of what Mr Serhal might say, and whether he'd think it was worth another shot. I'd come armed with all the information from the previous attempts – blood tests, reports, results, hospital notes etc., all organised by category in a black folder, in the hope that it would give him enough background to understand our situation. He probably thought I was crackers, but it was important for me to give as much history as possible so I would know I'd done everything I could.

I picked up a magazine but couldn't concentrate on reading it – even though it was quiet there was a lot going on with people being called and coming and going with files etc. Suddenly the room was fairly empty with only a couple of patients left waiting, then James appeared again and we were immediately called through to another consulting room.

Mr Serhal breezed in and my first impression of him was that he was quite a character! He seemed very boisterous and efficient, but very friendly and jolly too. He asked us to sit down then quickly skimmed through the file I'd brought with me. He was particularly interested in our first attempt that had worked then failed, and said that it was very rare for me to have been unlucky enough to get OHSS at that point. From my notes he couldn't see any reason why my physiology should point to that outcome.

He then asked James to pop behind the curtain so he could do a quick examination. As soon as he took a look he said, "Aah yes, that would be why you have a problem," which came as a complete surprise. Apparently James had a condition called varicocele, which is a widening of the veins in the testicles. It makes the temperature increase, impairing sperm production, and has an effect on quality. There's a lot of research to support this and, conversely, a lot of research that says having varicocele makes no difference whatsoever. In Mr Serhal's opinion though, and he'd obviously seen many patients before, it explained our problem.

I tried to take it in. Something so simple that gave us a reason – something that finally gave James an answer. Maybe he'd been wondering why all this time and now he knew. Maybe the reason wasn't relevant for him, but whatever he felt about it, there was actually an explanation. My mind turned back to the beginning of the investigations – why on earth hadn't this been discovered before in Oxford, and why hadn't James been examined properly right at the beginning? Not that it would've made any difference to the type of treatment necessarily, although I did know that it could sometimes be corrected by surgery. The thought of that would've sent James running for the hills though, so maybe it wouldn't have been an option anyway.

In the meantime Mr Serhal continued reading some of the test results that I'd given him, things like hormone levels etc., then he put the file down, looked straight at us and said that he thought he could definitely help us by doing a procedure called blastocyst transfer. Somewhere in my head a little voice shouted out loudly, "Yeeeees! He's thinking what I'm thinking!" I was right, blastocyst transfer *was* the right thing to do. Relief was definitely an understatement, and I realised there and then that this was the moment I'd been waiting for when I'd know which clinic was for us.

I looked at James briefly then turned to Mr Serhal and asked him when we could start what would be our last cycle. I knew it would cost us more than before but I had a really good feeling about it; that it was one hundred per cent the thing to do. There was even more good news – Mr Serhal said that given where I was in my menstrual cycle the timing was perfect and we could start treatment straight away. Wow. Everything had happened so fast, which was exactly how it should be. Not fast in a negative, worrying way, but absolutely, perfectly meant to be.

Mr Serhal continued to explain the ICSI cycle and told us the dates of what would happen when. It was a different protocol to the one we'd been used to in Oxford, but he explained that it was one that seemed to achieve good results overall. The first thing I had to do was to take the pill starting immediately, whilst I was still on the last few days of my menstrual cycle. This was considered to be around day four or five of the first part of the protocol. Then, sometime between days six and ten I had to return to the clinic so that a dummy embryo transfer could be performed, which would give the doctors an idea of how difficult or easy they could expect the real transfer to be. I also had to have something called a HyCoSy, or Hysterosalpingo-contrast-sonography – a visualisation of the endometrial cavity, uterus and sometimes the fallopian tubes by ultrasound scan. It was the proper name for the saline scan that I'd had before in Oxford. Both of these were scheduled for 13th April. Fifteen days later I'd start using the down-regulation spray, and three days after that I'd stop taking the pill. I'd have another menstrual period, then sometime during the first three days of my bleed I'd have a scan to check I was 'down-regulated', and if everything looked OK I'd start injecting the stimulating drugs. Four days later I'd have to return for a blood test, as well as having scans to check the progress of the ovaries on days seven, nine and eleven of injections. On day fourteen and after a final booster injection, I'd have egg collection, then five days later, after the eggs had been fertilised and the embryos were at blastocyst stage I'd have the embryo transfer. Then, once again and for the very last time, we'd have to wait.

I tried to take in the new way of doing things as it was all very different. This time I'd be scanned every other day as well as having additional blood tests, which was very encouraging. Of course, all of this had to be paid for – every single blood test, scan, and shot of drug, but the level of care seemed to be of a different world. I felt like a person, and I just knew that the clinic would do everything they could to make our last cycle a success.

I was brought back to the present by Mr Serhal's voice suggesting that I had a chlamydia swab and blood test for thyroid function there and then, followed by blood tests for James regarding chromosome studies, although given that he'd had them before we didn't expect the outcome to be any different. He then introduced us to some of the nursing staff and one of the other doctors led us away to a theatre where I had the chlamydia swab taken. We thanked Mr Serhal and he wished us all the best with the process. He wouldn't necessarily be involved in the egg collection or embryo transfer, but he assured us that all the staff were incredibly well qualified and we'd be in good hands.

Nearly two hours after our original appointment time we finally left the clinic. Our invoice to date totalled £657.50 and included fees for Microgynon 30 (the pill), Suprefact nasal spray (for down-regulation), chlamydia swab, chromosome studies, semen analysis, thyroid function test and the consultation with Mr Serhal. Our credit cards became very useful indeed!

As we left the building we were greeted by a wall of heavy rain; the bright day had turned into a dark sky, in complete contrast to my mood which had suddenly become the exact opposite. The unsettled sense of treading water until life kicked in again had disappeared and I allowed myself to hope. I looked at James and told him that I knew our decision to come to UCH had been the right one. I didn't dare wish for anything much so early on, but I knew we couldn't do any more than this, and that we wouldn't find a better clinic. The calm inside was a welcome feeling after the past couple of years of feeling completely lost.

Chapter 8

Third and Last

Thursday, 13th April 2006

Three days after our consultation I returned to the clinic for the dummy embryo transfer and HyCoSy. Events had moved on quickly giving me no time in which to mull things over, which was a good thing for me. I went to work a little earlier than normal in the morning, so I could leave just before 1 p.m., then it was the first of many mad dashes to the railway station in Didcot to catch a train for Paddington. I could've gone from Oxford but the trains weren't as regular and usually took a lot longer so I preferred to drive the small distance to catch a mainline train. I listened to Eros Ramazzotti on my car's CD player, as usual and probably at full volume, and sang my head off whilst driving down the A34. I actually felt quite lighthearted – it was a long time since I'd been acquainted with that feeling.

I parked my car then walked the short distance over the bridge to the station. I wanted to catch the 1.15 p.m. train, which would get me in to London at around 2 p.m., giving me an hour to get to UCH for my appointment at 3 p.m. I only had to wait a couple of minutes before it arrived so I boarded and made myself comfortable in a window seat, then took out my book and a 500ml bottle of water. I set myself the target of drinking the entire contents by the time we reached London – an embryo transfer is always done under abdominal sonogram, rather than an internal scan, and having a full bladder makes it easier to see the uterus. If I bought another 500ml bottle at Paddington station and drank all of that just before I reached the clinic I'd be fine. It wasn't particularly comfortable but it was necessary.

I read a few pages of my book, but couldn't really concentrate, so just ended up looking out of the window. It was a journey I came so used to taking, particularly towards the end of the stimulation part of the treatment, as I had to be in London pretty much every other day for a couple of weeks. It wasn't a lengthy journey though, and provided there were no hold-ups I didn't find it at all stressful.

Once I arrived at the station I decided to take a taxi to the clinic; time was a bit tight and I didn't want to risk missing my appointment. I walked through to the taxi rank where unusually there wasn't a queue so I had no problem getting a cab. I'd told James not to bother coming with me to all the appointments for scans etc. Given they were often during the afternoon we ended up meeting afterwards anyway so we could get something to eat at Ask in Spring Street near Paddington station before getting the train home.

The taxi driver took the back streets to Grey's Inn Road. I lost my bearings completely as it was a one-way system for a lot of the journey and it looked like we had to double back in order to go forward on several occasions. It was very quick though, and I arrived outside the front of the Eastman Dental Hospital with plenty of time to spare. I thanked and paid the driver then made my way through to the clinic. I didn't go through the main front door this time – there was a side entrance accessed through a rear courtyard that was slightly quicker, which the clinic had advised us to use in future.

The double doors opened automatically and I found myself directly in front of the reception area. It was 2.45 p.m. – I registered that I'd arrived with the receptionist, then sat down and took my book out again. I'd already finished the water I'd bought at the station so helped myself to another cup from the water dispenser – it wouldn't be long now so I was quite safe to top up, just to make sure. I did actually need to go to the bathroom already but I wanted the HyCoSy and dummy transfer to go without a hitch so I was happy to put up with feeling uncomfortable for just a little longer.

Well, 3 p.m. came, and went. As did 3.10 p.m., 3.15 p.m., and 3.20 p.m. I realised you had to allow for a certain level of delay, given the medical nature of it all, but I started to get anxious. Crossing and uncrossing my legs, I felt like a bit of an idiot. I tried to keep my mind on my book and just sat there, hoping it wouldn't be long. Another few minutes later at 3.30 p.m., I looked at the receptionist who promptly looked away again, having no idea how uncomfortable I was. I thought she'd forgotten I was waiting and debated with myself whether to risk getting out of my chair – a puddle on the floor not being a desired outcome!

I couldn't just sit there though, so the next time it was quiet, the phone wasn't ringing and she wasn't speaking to anyone else I decided I'd just get up and ask her what was going on. However, a minute or two later I was still sat there – I could see I wasn't going to get that chance, so the next time she looked up I fixed my eyes on her and gave her a 'hard stare'. It must have worked because she looked at me, got straight up and said that she'd just go and find out what the hold up was. Well thank goodness for that I thought as I whispered, "OK, thanks," then picked up a magazine and just stared at the pictures.

By this time it was getting on for 3.50 p.m. and I'd been waiting for an hour and five minutes. I honestly thought I was going to burst and I started panicking that either I'd get an infection from withholding, or that I couldn't have the exam because I wouldn't be able to hold on long enough. A couple of minutes later the receptionist returned and said that the doctor was just finishing with the last patient and then she'd be with me – no indication of a timescale though! I just had to sit and cross my fingers as well as my legs. It was very uncomfortable and I began to get really upset – thoughts of the Oxford hospital and how wrong everything went came back to me for a while. I closed my eyes and tried to focus on the reason why I was there, why I was putting myself through it one more time and to remember the positive feeling I'd had at our meeting with Mr Serhal the previous Friday.

I was forced back to the present by the sound of someone calling my name. I opened my eyes and saw a nurse with a clipboard in front of me – it was finally my turn. I stood up quickly and sighed. It was OK, I could hold on – now I knew they were ready it gave me something to concentrate on. The nurse smiled and told me to follow her through to theatre, all the time chatting away and apologising profusely for the long wait – apparently it was because they'd had a difficult dummy embryo transfer with the person before me. I completely understood but did wish they'd just told me that was the reason instead of letting me sit there thinking they'd forgotten about me. I'd started to worry about being delayed on egg collection day too, which was completely irrational probably, so I decided to ask a nurse later on about the chances of that happening.

Once in theatre the doctor explained that she'd do the dummy transfer first, then let me go to the bathroom so I'd be as comfortable as possible for the HyCoSy. The doctor and nurses were all so apologetic and kind about it too, and as there was no-one else after me they could take all the time they needed to ensure I was happy about everything. I couldn't believe what they were saying – I didn't expect that level of care and interest at all. I was so used to being one of many and feeling like just a number.

A nurse drew the curtain and asked me to undress from the waist down then I lay on the table and covered myself with the sheets. I looked at the ceiling and tried to relax. I'd been through it several times before so it didn't bother me at all, and was certainly no worse than having a cervical screening. During the procedure I chatted to one of the nurses about work and the weekend, and a couple of minutes later it was done, having shown up no problems whatsoever. I got off the bed and rushed to the ladies' – I'd never been so happy to see a toilet in my life!

Now that was out of the way and I could think properly my mind turned to the HyCoSy. Although I'd had one before it was still a bit daunting as the environment was so completely different. I made my way back to the theatre and lay down on the table again. I closed my eyes and tried to conjure up images of those tropical beaches for a second time – and it worked. I did feel some slight period-type pain when the fluid was injected through the catheter, but it didn't last long and the whole procedure was over in ten minutes or so. Apparently it was quite common to experience that same cramp-like pain, as well as some bleeding, during the hours that followed so I'd already taken a couple of paracetamol beforehand. Whilst rare, there was also a risk of infection so I was prescribed antibiotics, Metronidazole and Zithromax, just in case. Great, so not only had I been constantly prodded and poked by the doctors, I also had to take rectal suppositories!

I got myself dressed and made my way back to the waiting area, then a couple of minutes later I was called to the finance office to pay another invoice. I checked the printed sheet – two lots of antibiotics, £24; cervical swab, £65; HyCoSy procedure, £200; dummy embryo transfer, £90; making a total this time of £379. The running total to date was £1,036.50 – all in the space of a long weekend. I paid the bill and made my way back out on to Grey's Inn Road. I looked at my watch and saw that the time was coming up for 4.35 p.m. Now all I had to do was get home during rush hour which was completely unappealing. Maybe we could eat at Ask and catch a later train? It was way too much hassle competing with the hoards of commuters. I called James and told him that everything had gone alright and that I'd meet him at the office. We could go to Paddington together then, and decide about dinner on the way.

I decided to walk to Berkeley Square, so took a left turn and slowly made my way towards Oxford Street. From there it was another twenty-five minutes or so. As I walked I began to feel the expected cramp-like pain nagging away in my lower abdomen. My head though was strangely free of thoughts; it was as if there was a peaceful two or three week lull ahead, before I started using the first of the drugs. My confidence in UCH couldn't have been higher – they knew exactly what they were doing and I was happy with everything being in their hands. The only blot on the horizon was a small doubt about whether I'd be made to wait for any of the important procedures again, specifically on egg collection day. I decided to give one of the nurses a call – they said I could ring at any time if anything was bothering me, and if no-one was able to speak there and then they'd always call back, evenings and weekends included. I dialled the number on my mobile and spoke to the receptionist who put me on hold whilst she checked if anyone was available. Unfortunately no-one could speak to me, so I was transferred to the answerphone to leave a message. I garbled something about wanting to check a minor detail and that I'd appreciate a call back, then hung up.

I checked my watch again – 5.00 p.m. – I needed to get a move on in case we decided to eat before going home and wanted to get a table without having to wait an hour. I began to walk quite briskly, dodging the crowds of people on Oxford Street, and twenty minutes later I arrived in the lobby of James's office. After a short wait he appeared out of the lift then we grabbed a taxi and made our way to Paddington.

We decided it was definitely worth checking at Ask. It was the start of Easter weekend and incredibly busy, but the waiter found us a table for two fairly quickly, and after we'd ordered I checked my mobile to see if I'd missed any calls. There was an answerphone symbol showing, so I dialled in to retrieve it and to my annoyance it was one of the nurses at UCH – she must have called whilst we were in the taxi or something. She explained on the message that unfortunately, although the unit was open for collections and transfers, it was otherwise closed for the entire Easter weekend and someone would only be available the following Tuesday, unless it was an emergency. Feeling a bit discouraged I deleted the message and thought about what it was I wanted to ask the nurse anyway. Really, once I thought about it rationally, speaking to someone wouldn't change anything as there wasn't anything to change. It was just me being a bit paranoid as usual, and all I really needed from a nurse was reassurance. It wasn't going to make any difference whatsoever to the treatment or process so in the end I decided to let it go – it wouldn't have done me any good worrying about something that had already happened anyway, and I didn't want to ruin the weekend. I decided to log in to the Fertility Friends website later, or on Friday, and post a question to see if anyone else had experienced anything similar at UCH. In the meantime, I just enjoyed my pizza.

Friday, 14ᵗʰ April 2006

I posted my question on the fertility site forum then went out for the rest of the day. By the time I checked in the evening I'd had a couple of responses already. Apparently it was sometimes the case that appointments were unavoidably delayed somewhat, and it seemed that I'd just been unfortunate in experiencing it to that degree, given my full bladder. What did come across though was that the patients at UCH all raved about how professional and caring the unit was, and that they always called back regarding left messages, even if it was 10 p.m. I thought the best thing to do would be to factor in at least half an hour of lateness to any given appointment time – and to make sure I always took a book. Reassured, I was able to concentrate on having a peaceful weekend.

Sunday, 16th April 2006

My parents came down for Easter Sunday so we booked a table for lunch at Portobello in Summertown. The steaks and burgers were fantastic, and the homemade elderflower cordial with mint leaves was really lovely. For the rest of the time I just relaxed, read a book or two, watched TV a bit, and drank copious amounts of chai tea latte. I also had to remember to take the pill – something I hadn't done in a long time. The previous two protocols didn't involve taking it at all, and it was quite reassuring to be doing something a bit different this time.

Feeling incredibly positive I found myself willing the ten days by until I could start to use the down-regulation nasal spray, finally being able to let the process run its course without over-thinking every little detail. I was at the point of 'que sera sera' and it was liberating in a way. Of course, my whole mood could change within twenty-four hours so I made the most of my feeling of freedom.

Thursday, 20th April 2006

Just under a week later I started thinking about buying the drugs for injecting. I'd been told at the last appointment that I'd be using Menopur, a different drug to my other two cycles, and that it would require mixing first then injecting with a proper syringe, as opposed to the automatic pen device I'd been used to. The Fertility Friends forum came in useful yet again as I posted another question asking where other people had purchased their drugs from. They were sold by the ampoule and I needed at least twenty-two. I could buy them directly from UCH but apparently it was a very expensive way of doing it as they charged a supplement on top taking the cost to £21 per ampoule. A fellow patient suggested using a chemist in Shadwell who was able to supply the ampoules at £13 each, which meant a saving of £176. So that was a no brainer then – all I had to do was fax over my prescription once it had been issued and I could collect the day after, or they could be sent next day delivery to Oxford for £15 if it was easier. After some thought I decided that I'd probably prefer to go down to London to pick them up personally – I didn't fancy Parcelforce losing my precious parcel.

Thursday, 27th April 2006

Day one of the dreaded nasal spray arrived. I had to sniff once in each nostril four times per day, twice the amount that I'd had to do previously, so I decided on 7 a.m., 11 a.m., 7 p.m., and 11 p.m. I grabbed a carton of apple juice from the fridge and poured myself a small glass ready to drink immediately afterwards to try and mask the aftertaste. I thought I'd do it first, before breakfast and definitely before I cleaned my teeth. I also tried to remember to take my toothbrush in to work with me so I could do it again after the 11 a.m. spray.

Two quick sniffs and a glass of juice later I didn't feel too bad – clearly I was an expert by now. I also remembered that I had to take an aspirin, although there's some controversy surrounding whether it actually does any good or not, but some in the medical community believed it could help blood flow to the uterus. UCH advised a small dose of 75mgs daily as long as there were no reasons why it shouldn't be taken such as stomach ulcers or asthma. I didn't have any of those problems and as it wouldn't do any harm I decided to take it.

I took my last contraceptive pill on Sunday, 30th April and four days later I got my period. I called UCH to arrange an appointment for a scan to check that my ovaries were at baseline, and was booked in for the following day at 2.45 p.m.

Friday, 5th May 2006

I arrived at Paddington station and decided to take a taxi to the clinic and walk back – I hadn't been doing much exercise anyway as I'd reduced my gym visits, concerned as I was about overdoing things and making my body too tired. It was also very hot for a change and I thought it might cool down a bit for the return trip.

I got there in good time, and was surprised to find that I was called in for the scan straight away, where a very pleasant and softly spoken doctor said he'd be doing a vaginal ultrasound to check the ovaries. I'd had so many of those before that it didn't bother me at all and as he was very quick it was over in an instant. He confirmed that everything was as it should be and that I could start the injections that night. I was then sent downstairs, accessed by going outside into the courtyard and down some steps into what looked to be the basement but was actually the procedure area. After a short wait a friendly nurse took me into a small office type room and proceeded to show me how to mix the drugs and inject myself by demonstrating the process using that good old orange technique!

I had to mix powder with saline, then draw the fluid up into the syringe. After pinching together a small area on my abdomen I'd then inject myself with what seemed to be a huge needle. I was given the chance to practise on the orange, which I managed with no problem at all, then the nurse asked if I needed to purchase the drugs. I mentioned that I'd been given the prescription on my last visit and that I hoped to get it from the Shadwell pharmacy that some of the other patients at UCH had recommended. She told me that if I found there was a problem I could just let her know and they'd issue what I needed. I was also given a drug sheet that told me how much to inject and when, and on which dates I needed to return for scans and blood tests. That part was completely new; on previous cycles I'd only had one scan nearly three quarters of the way through injecting. It was good to know that I'd be monitored so closely and that they really wanted to get the drug dosage perfectly right to give me the best chance of success in terms of egg maturity. It also helped put my mind at rest with regard to over-stimulating and getting OHSS again.

I made my way back up the steps and out into the courtyard. I didn't have an invoice to pay this time as the scans for treatment were included in the main fees. I made my way out to Grey's Inn Road and started walking towards Chancery Lane tube station, where I could connect to Bank then change on to the DLR to Shadwell.

Half an hour later I stepped onto Shadwell platform and walked down the steps. I think something had happened, or was about to, as there were several policemen at the entrance to the station and whilst the pharmacy was apparently only around the corner, I started to feel a little uncomfortable and just wanted to get there, then get back on the train. I'd been given directions to turn left out of the station and continue walking straight on until I approached a main road; the pharmacy should then be on my left-hand side near the junction.

After walking for a few minutes I spotted a blue pharmacy sign so went in and headed straight for the counter. I'd already faxed over the prescription a couple of days before so I hoped it was ready for me to pick up. I told the guy behind the counter my name and as he went off to find my package I turned around and spotted a fridge with various drinks on display. It was still ridiculously hot and I felt really thirsty so I grabbed a bottle of water just as he put my parcel of drugs on the counter. Twenty-two ampoules of Menopur and associated mixing fluid and syringes equalled £286 on the credit card. I said I'd pay cash for the bottle of water but he just waved at me and said that I could have it, no need to pay. I was taken aback as it was really unexpected and I was very grateful. I would always remember that small gesture of kindness.

I put the prescription in a canvas bag that I always kept folded up in my handbag then made my way to the tube station. I didn't have long to wait before a train arrived and as I sat down on the way back to Bank I thought I may as well keep going on the tube rather than walk. Whilst it would be quite stifling in the underground at least I wouldn't have to fight with the hordes of people down Oxford Street.

As usual I was supposed to be meeting James at Paddington and when I walked into the main station saw that it was only 4.30 p.m. – I still had an hour and a half to wait. I called him and we agreed that I'd just get the next train home. He still had a bit of work to do and I needed to make sure I wasn't too late as I had to do my injection in the evening.

I picked up a chai tea latte then browsed in the concourse store windows whilst I waited for the next train at 5 p.m. I thought how amazing it was that women could always seem to find the smallest window of opportunity in which to shop, as I boarded the train with a Monsoon carrier bag in my hand!

I arrived back home just before 6 p.m. then made a cup of tea and tried to relax. Things were always worse when I was on my own in the apartment. It brought back memories of what had happened before and I sometimes found it difficult to be alone in complete silence. I put the TV on for company then prepared some mushroom risotto – it was one of my favourites and James didn't really like rice so I often made it whenever I ate alone. By the time I'd finished and put everything in the dishwasher it was getting on for 7.30 p.m. My instructions from the clinic had been to start the stimulation injections this evening, at some point after 7 p.m. It had to be at the same time every day so I plumped for 8 p.m. – time enough to finish dinner and load the dishwasher.

I read through the information leaflet as I repeated the

instructions the nurse had given me – I had to mix two capsules of powder with one dose of saline then suck up the fluid using a detachable green needle. Once all the fluid was in the syringe I had to change the needle to the brown one, ready for injecting. I knew that the first time I did it I'd be a bit worried in case I messed up mixing the fluid. I had a 'proper' syringe to inject with this time and the needle was awfully long, especially compared to the short click pen I'd been used to.

I took the syringe, attached the correct needle and drew up the required amount of saline solution. I then snapped off the tops of two vials of the Menopur and pierced the seal of one of them, injecting the saline down into the powder. I gently swirled the vial to mix the fluid, then turned it upside down and drew the solution back in to the syringe, which was still attached. So far so good. As I'd been told to use two powders to one measure of saline I did the same again with the second vial, using the solution I'd just mixed with the first powder. Drawing this new fluid back up into the syringe I then discarded the empty vials into the sharps bin that the clinic had given me, detached the mixing needle and attached the new one for injecting. I tapped the top of the syringe to ensure any bubbles were at the top, then very gently pushed the plunger until a small drop of fluid appeared at the end of the needle. Taking an alcohol swab I wiped the injection site on my abdomen, then pinched an inch of skin together and braced myself! I'd decided not to bother with ice; several patients on the Fertility Friends website had said that it made no difference anyway and it was just another thing to faff about with. I held the syringe like a pencil, took a deep breath and pushed the needle into my skin at a forty-five degree angle.

OK, that wasn't so bad. I pushed down on the syringe and watched the small amount of fluid disappear, then retracted the needle, disposed of the syringe in the sharps bin and put the medication back in the fridge. I looked at the site where I'd just injected and it already looked a bit on the red side and was beginning to sting slightly. The clinic had told me that it was possible to have visible side effects such as redness or bruising, especially after so many days using the same injection site. Their advice was to alternate it; to one day use the left side of my abdomen, then the next use the right. The whole thing had taken no more than five minutes and I surprised myself about how not bothered I'd been. I had to do exactly the same for the next two nights, then return to the clinic for a scan and a blood test. Feeling exceptionally calm and collected I settled down to watch TV for the rest of the evening, looking forward to a quiet weekend.

Monday, 8th May 2006

I had the day off today as my clinic appointment was at 11 a.m. I'd finally got round to telling some of my other work colleagues, and everyone who knew was really understanding. I told my managers that I'd work a couple of full days later on to make up for the time.

When I got to Didcot station I bought a weekly railcard – it was the least expensive option as I had to go to UCH at least every other day for a week. I arrived in London at around 10.15 a.m., picked up a chai tea latte as usual then took a taxi over to the clinic. I had twenty minutes to spare when I got to reception so pulled out my book and tried to read. It felt a little strange to be back again so soon. I was still trying to get used to the intensity of the cycle, with all the double strength sniffing, monitoring and regular blood tests – they certainly looked after their patients well.

I heard my name being called and looked up to see a doctor with a clipboard in her hand; it was my turn for a scan. Suddenly my stomach flipped and the nerves kicked in. It was the first scan since starting the injections and I didn't really know what they expected to see so early on. The doctor led me to a small scan room and I hopped on to the examination table whilst she proceeded to tell me that she'd be doing a transvaginal scan. I removed my lower clothing then covered myself with the blanket and lay back. I could see the screen to my right, and as the doctor began I slowly managed to relax. After a couple of minutes she told me that everything looked fine, although the levels of a hormone called E2 had to be checked to see if the dose of Menopur needed to be increased – my ovaries were still on the small side.

At this early stage it didn't mean anything but at least if they did have to increase it they could ease off a little later on in the week if necessary, rather than worry about leaving it until later when there may not be enough time. I was a bit disappointed to be honest and wondered why nothing much had happened. I'd done three injections already so surely they should have had an effect? Trying to compare with my last cycles was impossible – I only had one scan more than halfway through the stimulation part so I didn't know how I'd progressed at the same stage previously. I wondered whether it was such a good idea to know so much so early on; maybe it would just make me anxious?

On the other hand, and like the doctor said, if they

found that suddenly things took off due to the increased Menopur then it would be easier to reduce it down later rather than have a last minute panic and have to do it the other way around. I tried to tell myself not to think so much about it, although inevitably it was in the back of my mind – how I wished I wasn't such a worrier.

I got dressed then made my way into the courtyard outside and down the stairs to the procedure area in the basement where a nurse was waiting to take my blood. I'd had that many tests by now that all my good veins had started to collapse and it was sometimes difficult to locate the right spot. After a short wait to get the test straight back from the lab the level of E2 hormone was confirmed at around the 170 mark. It was slightly lower than expected and the decision was to up my dose of Menopur from 150iu to 225iu for the next two days. I was also told to stop using the Suprefact sniffing spray as it could be that it suppressed the stimulation drugs too much. A review would be done again after my Wednesday appointment.

Trying not to let this small hiccup bother me I made my way up the basement stairs then popped back to reception to arrange my appointment time for two days later. Feeling deflated I made my way back to Paddington as I wanted to get back home as soon as possible. I started to get a hollow sensation in my stomach and, recognising it was stress, I tried to still my mind but the traffic noise and sheer amount of people made it impossible. I chided myself as I realised it was no good worrying about the lack of follicular activity. That was why the doctor had upped the dosage. For some reason I had the idea in my head that everything would go perfectly and I'd be quite mellow all the way through, although that was obviously rather an unrealistic expectation. UCH knew what they were doing though and no-one appeared to be concerned. In fact it was probably quite normal – a slow start that would pick up later on. I knew that once I arrived back home I'd feel a bit better; I could sleep for a while, or listen to some music.

At Paddington station I checked the departures board and luckily there was a train due to leave fifteen minutes later. I bought a bottle of water from WHSmith then checked myself in through the barrier and found a seat on the train. I began to think about the Fertility Friends website and the comments I'd read recently from a few patients who had been to either UCH or the ARGC, about an acupuncturist in Harley Street. After my previous experiences of acupuncture I didn't know whether to give it another go or not. I decided to phone and see if I could speak to someone about how often and when during the cycle they suggested treatment. I thought I might have left it a bit late but I could always call and find out. My head had been given something else to think about and I began to feel a bit more cheerful. I closed my eyes for a while and the next thing I knew the train was pulling into Didcot railway station. Half an hour later I was home so I switched on my laptop and waited for it to fire up whilst I made myself a cup of tea. I had to find out the number for the acupuncture clinic so logged on to Fertility Friends and searched for the thread that mentioned the details.

It was called The London Acupuncture Clinic and it seemed to be the only one that offered a seven day a week service during embryo transfer for IVF patients. There were some incredibly good reviews of how helpful they are and they apparently had a star acupuncturist called Daniel Elliott. To be honest I think my mind was made up already. The clinic wasn't too far from UCH so access wouldn't be a problem, and given the amount of money we'd already spent a little bit extra to help my peace of mind was definitely worth it.

I dialled the number and after a couple of rings a pleasant sounding lady answered. I explained that I was a patient at UCH and that I'd heard Daniel provided a service for IVF cycles. She told me that he did indeed do this and that he usually recommended a double appointment on the day of embryo transfer – just beforehand and directly afterwards. I decided to go ahead and book the appointment – I'd already been given a date in two weeks' time for the transfer, assuming the blastocyst stage had been successful, so she pencilled my name in the diary, and said that I just needed to advise on the exact timing as soon as I knew. I thanked her and put the phone down. My mood lifted – I was happy that I'd managed to get that sorted. After reviewing the website and checking out credentials, along with those of previous IVF patients I knew I'd made the right decision.

Wednesday, 10th May 2006

As I sat in the waiting room once again I began to think about whether the increased dose of stimulation drug would have had any effect. I'd only injected two days' worth; would it really make that much difference already? It didn't take me long to find out as I was soon called in to the scan room. Some mouse clicking and recording of results later, the doctor told me I had eight follicles and my E2 hormone level was at 680. That sounded a bit on the low side again to me. I asked what they would have expected at this point but unfortunately there was no right answer. Those that were there were of the expected size, and I should have known by now that the amount of follicles had no bearing on the amount of potential eggs.

Still, it was rather disappointing once again and I left the clinic in a sad state of mind. The doctor had given me instructions to up the dose again to five ampoules and to return in two days' time for another scan, but told me that it was nothing to be concerned about. I decided to walk back to the station again, as it would give me some time to think things through and try and force myself to be rational and positive. To be honest I was a bit fed up with hearing the word 'positive', as if that would have any bearing on the outcome. Damn annoying being told that all the time. I was also worn out by all my mood swings; one minute I was sad, the next I'd talked myself into being upbeat. I didn't know if I was coming or going.

By the time I'd reached the station the thought of the lack of follicles and having to stop sniffing the spray still bothered me so I decided to give the clinic a ring to try and put my mind at rest. I managed to get through to a nurse straight away and explained my worries. She was lovely and completely understood why I was so anxious. She mentioned that they could do a blood test for levels of LH (luteinising hormone), which is an accurate predictor of ovulation, and if it looked like it was imminent they could bring forward egg collection, or give less of the booster shot at the end. She arranged to do the test on Friday when I was next due at the clinic.

I also tried my best to adopt a 'what will be will be' frame of mind, which did help somewhat, if only for a while. Anyway, I had something else to think about – funds! I had to buy more stimulation drugs as the original batch I'd purchased from Shadwell had nearly run out given my dosage had been increased several times. I'd been given another prescription from the clinic so stopped by the pharmacy attached to my local doctors' surgery in Oxford to see if they had it in stock or whether I had to place an order. I was in luck – they had enough in to last me a couple of days and assured me that they'd order the remainder for me to collect on Friday. I assumed that my dose would be increased again so ordered more than I needed just to make sure. The expense of all the extras kept mounting up but there was nothing I could do and at that point I just didn't care.

Friday, 12th May 2006

Friday came around quickly – where did Thursday go? I was grateful for the fact that I had some work to do in between clinic appointments as it helped to keep my mind off things. I went into work for an hour, then left to get the train from Didcot at around 10 a.m. I'd arrive in London a bit early but didn't want to risk the train being late and missing my appointment. I sat in a window seat and closed my eyes. I'd begun to feel a little tired what with all the journeys in and out of London, and the stress of wondering what was happening to my body and whether it was doing what it should be doing at this point. I must have nodded off as the next thing I heard was the tannoy announcement saying we'd be arriving in London in the next couple of minutes.

Once the train stopped at the platform I waited for everyone else to move before getting up from my seat. I made my way up the platform to the main concourse, then checked my watch and realised I had enough time to stop at Starbucks for my usual. Cup in hand, I joined the queue at the taxi rank and after a couple of minutes was in a cab weaving its way through the back streets to get to the clinic. It was busy with quite a few roadworks still and we had to follow a diversion or two, but eventually I arrived with time to spare.

I paid the driver then walked under the arch and through the courtyard to the rear entrance. After registering at reception I was sent downstairs for the blood tests first, as the doctors were a little bit behind with their schedule. Eventually though it was my turn for a scan and I felt my insides start to churn again. That familiar old feeling of expectation had returned.

I made myself comfortable on the table and waited for the doctor. He breezed in all smiley and cheerful, and proceeded to do the scan. Follicles were still not too numerous but the contents were of a perfect size and quantity. He suggested increasing the dose by one more vial of powder over the weekend to maximise the chances of any additional maturing follicles. I had to return on the Monday morning for a final review before the plan for egg collection could be confirmed. With a sigh I dressed quickly then made my way back to the station and home.

Once back in our apartment I remembered to organise a hotel room for the following Wednesday night – the evening before what would hopefully be egg collection day. I had to be at the clinic's theatre reception at 8 a.m., so we were going to stay in London and just get a taxi that morning. The last thing I needed was stress about having to get up and catch a train from Didcot so early, worrying about whether it would be cancelled or delayed.

I knew of a comfortable hotel called The White House near Regent's Park which was perfect and not too far away from Grey's Inn Road, so I called reservations and booked us in. The flexible rate meant that if I had to change the date to the day after or before then it wouldn't be a problem.

With that sorted and nothing else urgent to do I had a relaxing weekend ahead of me; as far as that was possible given the circumstances. The countdown to egg collection day was getting shorter, and with it my memories of what had been before. It was still difficult to completely stop negative thoughts from clouding my head but I was grateful that this last cycle and everything about it was so different, and found myself unfamiliarly focused, calm, and full of optimism.

Monday, 15th May 2006

It was final scan day and my appointment was another early one – 10.30 a.m. So far I hadn't experienced any side effects, specifically pain and bloating, which meant that my body hadn't over-reacted to the drugs. Then again, the first time round I didn't have any symptoms either until after embryo transfer. I kept telling myself to have faith in the cycle – surely the odds were in our favour this time?

I was called through for the scan fairly quickly – everything looked to be as it should, and after another blood test and check for LH, I was given an instruction sheet about preparing for egg collection. That night

I had to inject the last dose of stimulation drug followed by 10,000iu of booster shot the evening after at 8 p.m. Wednesday would be a drug-free day, then it would be nil by mouth from midnight, apart from a small amount of water before 6 a.m. the next morning. The egg collection appointment was put in the diary for 9 a.m. on Thursday, 18th May 2006.

With the first stage behind me, I adopted a living in the moment attitude and tried to relax as much as possible so that I'd be ready for Thursday. Strangely it felt as though I was an observer rather than an active participant, which I thought was a good thing as it prevented me from being 'in my head' all the time. As I stepped outside the clinic the sun was shining, the sky was perfectly clear and for a brief moment something inside me said that it would all be OK.

Wednesday, 17th May 2006

It was my last day at work for a couple of weeks. I finished at my usual time of 1 p.m., then drove back home to pack an overnight bag for our stay in London. I took a dressing gown and slippers for theatre on Thursday and some loose fitting clothes to go home in afterwards. I had some linen trousers somewhere so I dug them out and thought I'd travel down in them too so I wouldn't need to take a spare pair. I put the rest of my things in the bag then called for a taxi to take me to Oxford station – I didn't want to leave my car overnight at Didcot, and whilst the journey from Oxford was a bit longer it was more convenient this time. As I sat in the taxi I watched the buildings go by down Abingdon Road. It felt good to be leaving Oxford for the London clinic, almost as if the slate had been wiped clean.

Once at Paddington station I took another taxi to James's office, then after half an hour or so we made our way to the hotel. We dropped our bags in the room then went in search of a decent restaurant for an early dinner – I needed to make sure I got enough rest as we had to be up quite early on Thursday morning.

Afterwards we headed back to the hotel where I tried to read my book for a while. The minutes ticked by on the clock, and as the hours flew and the time for our very last chance got nearer my head began to think too much. Compared to before I was actually quite composed and not particularly worried about the procedure, although I was completely aware that could all change by morning.

Thursday, 18th May 2006

I woke up early after a restless night. It had been too hot in the room and not only had I been unable to stop myself from focusing on the hum of the air conditioning units on the roof, my mind had also gone into overdrive trying to process that this really was the last time – if it didn't work I knew that I wouldn't have the strength to go through it all again, never mind the financial implications.

As the clock nudged nearer to 7.30 a.m. we collected our bags and went downstairs to reception where a taxi waited to take us the short journey to the clinic. It was already busy with traffic and commuters but in no time at all we arrived at the hospital and made our way straight downstairs to the theatre unit. One of the nurses showed us to a curtained cubicle containing a bed and a chair then, after I'd made myself comfortable, a doctor came to chat to us to make sure I was happy about the procedure.

There was another lady about to go into theatre, but after that it would be my turn so I sat on the bed and began to change into the hospital gown, my dressing gown and slippers. I'd just settled back on to the bed when one of the nurses approached and said I could have something to eat after the procedure, then asked me what I'd like in my sandwich. I was stunned into silence for a brief moment, as if I'd misheard what she'd said. Sandwich? Really? And I had a choice? It was like being in a hotel!

James and I chatted for a while as we waited for the other patient before me to return. After twenty minutes or so the door opened and she was brought back into the ward area in a wheelchair. I tried to still the increasing anxiety by taking deep breaths, as it dawned on me that I was next. Reality kicked in, and with it the comprehension that this really was it. If there weren't enough good eggs then it was game over. Luckily I didn't have much time to dwell on those thoughts as the nurse came through and asked me to follow her to theatre. It was a proper theatre environment and no-one else was allowed to sit in, so James gave me a quick kiss and I disappeared off through the double doors.

I opened my eyes slowly and saw James sitting in a chair next to the bed. I was a bit woozy and felt like I wanted to sleep, but I tried to wake myself up sufficiently to speak as a nurse came into view round the other side of the bed and asked me how I felt. Once I'd opened my eyes a bit more my head started to clear and the room slowly came into focus. I tried to sit and someone propped me up on some pillows. It felt weird, almost like floating, which was a completely new sensation – perhaps they'd used more or different sedative to the Oxford clinic.

I turned to James and said that I could do with a cup of tea. Ten minutes later the drugs must have worn off as I was totally lucid and feeling ravenous. A nurse appeared round the side of the curtain with a mug of tea and a plate of sandwiches. She told me that everything had gone well and that a doctor would come and talk to us about the outcome shortly. We didn't have to wait long before he appeared and confirmed what the nurse had said; that everything had gone to plan, they hadn't encountered any problems and that they'd retrieved twenty eggs.

I was stunned into complete silence. Twenty? How was that possible given how many follicles I'd had? It was getting on for double the amount than before. I was completely amazed. Of course, it didn't mean that they were all good quality but the fact that we had so many to start with was fantastic. We just had to wait to see how many fertilised, then how many would make it to the blastocyst stage. Still, one thing at a time – we'd done really well so far.

The doctor said that I could go as soon as I was able to walk adequately, so I swung my legs round the bed and attempted the short distance to the bathroom. Wow, that ached. My abdomen felt as if it had been continuously punched; it was so, so sore. It was probably because there'd been a lot more eggs and it had taken longer to get to them all.

I managed to hobble to the bathroom and back and another half hour or so later, after instructions to begin using progesterone pessaries that evening, the doctor gave me the all clear to go home. First, though, there was the small matter of payment to attend to so we made our way back up the steps and into the main building to the clinic's small admin office behind reception. I fished my credit card out of my bag then looked at the invoice – £3,770. Eek. That was a lot of money. It wasn't unexpected though, and as I waited for my card to be authorised I found myself contemplating how on earth we'd pay it all back, although that was completely irrelevant; we'd find a way. By the time we'd finished with the paperwork in the office it was nearly lunchtime so we took a taxi straight to Paddington station. I wanted to get home as quickly as possibly – the physical effects of the procedure had started to settle in and I was so tired that the only place I wanted to be was in my own bed.

I stared at the ceiling. My abdomen was really painful. I'd taken a couple of painkillers as soon as we'd arrived home but they hadn't really done anything and I could feel myself getting worked up. For some reason my emotions were suddenly all over the place. My head hurt and I just wished I could be knocked out for a few days so I didn't have to think. I glanced at the clock beside the bed and saw that it was late evening; at least I'd managed to sleep for a few hours. I got up to go to the bathroom by slowly swinging my legs to the side of the bed and grabbing on to the corner posts to guide me round to the ensuite. My whole body was so heavy and my head felt like it was swimming. I washed my hands then slowly shuffled back to my side of the bed again. I couldn't move very fast at all – the aching pain was just unbearable.

As I sat back down I could feel myself getting upset for what seemed like no reason whatsoever. I started to take some deep breaths; then even deeper breaths; then it felt like I couldn't breathe at all. I called out to James several times whilst trying to take in huge gulps of air.

"Oh no," I thought. "Please don't let me have OHSS again." My chest hurt and I couldn't breathe properly – what was happening? James rushed in and between the chest pains I garbled that I had to get to the hospital; I thought there was something wrong with my lungs and I felt dizzy, like I was going to lose consciousness.

With my heart pounding I slowly made it down the apartment staircase and into the car. James drove us out of the driveway at speed, wheels spinning in the gravel. I tried to take deep breaths but couldn't – all I could manage were short, quick gasps and I began to get somewhat hysterical. After what felt like a very long journey we arrived at the hospital car park. James helped me walk to the A&E department where he began to register my arrival at the reception desk. I just stood there like an idiot, trying to speak one word sentences in between my tears, "Can't. Breathe. Hurts. Help."

The receptionist told us to sit and wait at which point James ordered her to get someone there and then. He explained I'd had IVF egg collection that morning and I clearly couldn't breathe! To say he was furious was an understatement. It must have worked because a minute later someone rushed over with a wheelchair and I was taken off to triage. I somehow managed to haul myself up on to the bed, and a doctor came straight over to see what the problem was.

She took one look at me then said she wasn't going to examine me until I'd calmed down. What? Calmed down? I couldn't damn well breathe, you daft woman! I looked at her astonished, then she handed me a paper bag, told me to inhale deeply into it, and explained that I was having a rather severe panic attack. James tried to coach me into breathing in a controlled manner, but it took some time before I managed it. I couldn't focus as my chest hurt badly every time I took a breath. I really tried hard to concentrate – I just wanted the pain to stop.

After a few more minutes I felt the urgency slow down to something that resembled near normal. The pain in my chest eased and I could finally breathe normally so the doctor returned to have a chat. I told her that I'd just been through a third round of IVF/ICSI and that today had been egg collection day. I explained that on a previous attempt I'd got OHSS and had found it hard to breathe, so I'd thought that the same thing was happening again. She said that I was probably very anxious given the soreness and pain I was in, and that it may have prompted me to panic, resulting in the attack. The problem with a panic attack is that once it starts there isn't much you can do to stop it apart from try to focus and let it take its course. It was usually over within thirty minutes but it's possible to have several in succession, which was probably what had happened. With my breathing back to normal and my blood pressure checked, the doctor said I could go. By the time we got back home I was completely drained. Upset, in pain, and with an army of pillows to prop me up and as many painkillers as I was allowed, I finally managed to sleep.

Saturday, 20th May 2006

I spent most of Friday sleeping, resting and reading. My abdomen was still very sore and painful and I didn't feel like doing much at all. The clinic had rung on the Friday morning to say that out of the twenty eggs fertilised, we'd lost only five subsequent embryos overnight. I knew that was normal so at that point I wasn't overly concerned, and I couldn't do anything about it anyway.

By morning when the clinic rang again, ten embryos were doing great, three hadn't survived, and two were developing too quickly. The blastocyst transfer was planned for five days after the egg collection day on Tuesday, 23rd May. We just hoped that at least one embryo survived and would be of good enough quality to transfer.

Just before midday the soreness had worn off sufficiently for me to walk without being too uncomfortable, so we decided to do what we usually did at the weekend, trying to create as normal an environment as possible. I thought the familiarity of routine would help me to relax, so we went into Oxford for lunch, after which I spent the rest of the afternoon sitting in Borders bookshop, drinking a chai tea latte and reading the magazines. I tried not to think too much, although I inevitably failed. I found myself wondering how the remaining embryos were doing. The clinic gave us an update on a daily basis, even on Sunday, and each time I had to try and focus on being in the moment rather than fast-forwarding to what would happen the next day.

Sunday, 21st May 2006

As Sunday arrived and the call came through early in the morning, we learned that two embryos hadn't survived the night, but that we still had eight progressing nicely. We'd arranged to meet our friends Anna and Chris for lunch as we had to talk about the plan and timings for Tuesday. Anna said she'd drive me to London, be with me at the embryo transfer, and drive me back home again. Unfortunately my mum was unable to get to Oxford until late afternoon as she was working and I told James that he didn't need to take more time off work either. It would be quite a chaotic day – I had acupuncture appointments both before and after the transfer, and there was no telling how long everything would take. It would be a case of just going with the flow and trying not to get stressed about it.

Monday, 22nd May 2006

After quite a restful night and only a small amount of soreness remaining, we received the early morning update call – as the embryos developed further the risk of losing them increased, and that's exactly what had happened overnight. We still had four good embryos, with the other four still doing 'OK', whatever that meant. With only one more day to go before embryo transfer, even if we lost fifty per cent overnight we should still be able to transfer at least one. My hopes rose steadily. If we could transfer one or two blastocyst embryos then I'd know we'd done all that we could possibly do and whilst it would be a tense two week wait afterwards my mind and my heart were at the point of acceptance.

Tuesday, 23rd May 2006

Anna picked me up around 9 a.m. so we could get to London in plenty of time. I was really grateful to her for helping me, and told her that the least I could do was pay for petrol and treat her to lunch, especially as she was giving up her time to be with me.

It was a bright day and the sun was trying to make

an appearance, and as we drove down the M40 towards London we chatted about this and that, trying to keep the mood light-hearted. It started to get quite busy with traffic as we reached the outskirts of the city, but as Anna was used to driving into London for work it didn't take us long to arrive in Marylebone.

We parked the car and made our way to the restaurant. I'd managed to find one in Marylebone called Eat and Two Veg which served organic food. It was perfect as it was only a quick drive away from both the acupuncturist on Harley Street and the clinic. By the time we arrived I was ravenous so I ordered vegetarian sausage and mash with copious amounts of gravy. It was so good – real comfort food. In between mouthfuls Anna asked me if I was getting nervous. Surprisingly, I wasn't. I knew the transfer wasn't at all painful or uncomfortable, and as I hadn't heard anything from the clinic I assumed that there was at least one embryo to transfer.

We finished our meal in good time so I ordered a peppermint tea and Anna had a cappuccino, but we both declined pudding as we were completely full. I was due at the clinic at 2.00 p.m. and my half hour acupuncture appointment was at 1.00 p.m. Drinking the last of my tea I checked my watch and saw that it was 12.45 p.m. – just enough time to drive round to Harley Street. Anna dropped me off in front of the building; she'd come back to wait for me once she'd found the car park round the corner. I walked up the steps and into the reception area, then I was taken straight to the treatment room. I made myself comfortable and a couple of minutes later Daniel came in.

We'd not met in person before and after a brief

introduction he sat down and asked me how I felt. I told him that it felt odd, almost as if it was someone else that I was observing rather than it being me. I thought for a moment then realised that I was actually very calm, but excited at the same time. It was quite a good state to be in given the circumstances, although it did take a huge amount of focus to stay in such a positive mindset. It was the most important stage of the most important treatment cycle, and probably the most important experience of my life. Looking at it like that though would've been enough to send anyone round the bend, so I tried to just 'get on with it' without thinking too much.

Anyway, Daniel proceeded to insert the needles into the different points, then told me to just close my eyes and try and empty my mind, and that he'd return fifteen minutes later. Needless to say, emptying my mind was nigh on impossible – try as I might I couldn't banish my thoughts. I didn't yet know for sure how many, if any, embryos we had to transfer, and the thought of the impending transfer procedure, whilst not painful, was ever present. I tried to relax nonetheless, in between taking sips of water from a two litre bottle that I'd brought with me. A full bladder was necessary for the transfer this time as it made it easier to see all the internal organs apparently. I'd also taken a Cyclogest pessary first thing that morning, as well as a Voltarol pessary, an anti-inflammatory drug, two hours before the transfer was due. Cyclogest is a progesterone hormone and I had to take it every day until the pregnancy test.

As I relaxed I started to go through a mental checklist of everything I'd had to do with respect to the transfer, such as removing my nail varnish and remembering not to wear any perfume, not that I wore it much anyway. By the time I'd finished reviewing everything Daniel returned. That was quick – I looked at my watch and saw that it was 1.30 p.m. A couple of minutes later, after all the needles had been removed, Daniel ushered me out of the room. He said a cheerful goodbye and that he'd see me in a couple of hours. He told me that my appointment would be open indefinitely for the day, so even if I was late they wouldn't be going home until I'd been back for my final treatment. They were obviously used to seeing patients at all hours of the day, and it was heartening knowing that they really did care about their patients. I popped my head round the door of reception to tell Anna I was ready then we made our way to the car park in one of the adjacent streets. There were twenty minutes left in which to get to Grey's Inn Road – plenty of time.

Anna turned into the clinic's courtyard where we'd been given a permit to park for a few hours. We had to allow an hour and a half for the transfer, just in case it was held up for any reason. We made our way down the stairs to the theatre area where a nurse showed us to a bed at the far end of the ward. I hadn't really noticed the room much when I'd had the egg collection procedure. It was small and had a homely feel, with only eight or so beds each separated by a curtain. Several of them were occupied by other patients. Apparently they were running a bit late, although this wasn't as critical for transfers as it was for egg collections.

I changed into a theatre gown then one of the nurses asked me if I'd drunk enough water. I told her that I'd had about a litre so far so there shouldn't be any problem.

However, they still scanned my abdomen to make sure my bladder was full enough, and I was surprised to be told that I needed to drink some more. Apparently my uterus hadn't been pushed into the optimal position for transfer. I panicked a bit. There was no way I could fit any more liquid in without bursting, but fit it in I must. I returned to my bed and proceeded to gulp down as much water as possible. After half an hour or so I was rescanned but, unfortunately, nothing had changed.

The nurses looked a bit confused given the amount of liquid I'd drunk so far, but after waiting a little longer the doctors decided to take me through to theatre anyway. I made myself as comfortable as I could on the bed, then one of the female doctors came to speak to me. She said that we had two very good quality blastocyst embryos to transfer. Two blastocysts – my chances of a successful cycle had just increased dramatically. Hope surged and whilst I tried to remain calm I found myself getting all worked up again, but not, this time, in a bad way. It was more of an excited feeling of anticipation; or at least it would be once they'd managed to do the transfer.

The doctor began one more scan, which revealed that my uterus still wasn't adequately visible. She explained that they'd have to insert a catheter so I could be filled up artificially. I looked at Anna, who'd been allowed in to the transfer theatre with me, and clearly my face must have betrayed my feelings of horror at the thought. I could feel tears pricking my eyes. Why couldn't it all just fall into place without any problems? Anna took my hand and asked me if I was OK. She tried to reassure me, saying that it was alright, it would work out. The doctor reappeared to tell me that it would be a little uncomfortable for a short while when they inserted the catheter, but that once it was in place there wouldn't be any pain and I wouldn't be able to feel anything. I nodded resignedly. Maybe the look on my face changed her mind as she paused for a moment seeming to reconsider, then she said that they'd try one more thing first – tipping the bed so that my head was pointing slightly backwards and down towards the floor. Sometimes that made the internal organs move around a little and it was worth a try. She completely understood how stressful it was becoming for me, with what felt like an absolutely full bladder. Never mind the embryo transfer, all I could focus on was the fact that I badly needed the bathroom and no-one believed me!

The doctor pressed a button and the bed slowly tipped, then she began one last scan. I stared at her nervously, trying to work out what she was seeing on the screen from the look in her eyes. Suddenly she smiled, then said that it looked as though they wouldn't need to use a catheter after all – as predicted, moving my body by that small amount had shifted things around inside slightly and they could now quite clearly see my completely full to bursting bladder, and a perfect view of my uterus. My whole body visibly relaxed. It was going to be alright after all.

The transfer procedure began straight away, and the doctor brought my attention to the monitor screen mounted high on the wall to my left. Once the tube had been inserted into my uterus they'd slowly transfer the embryos. If I kept my eye on the monitor I'd be able to see a magnified image of the two blastocysts before they moved them down into the transfer catheter. I looked at the screen and waited for a few moments. Suddenly, there they were. I couldn't believe my reaction. I just grinned and my eyes began to water. My insides flipped and for a moment time stood still. I looked at Anna who was grinning with me. Seeing them before they were transferred made the whole thing so real, so personal. Did I feel happy, excited, worried, anxious, calm, or what? I had no idea – it was such a mix of feelings.

I nodded to say I was ready and then they were gone from the screen and were on their way to their final destination. Two minutes later and that was it, transfer done. One of the nurses said I could get up and go to the bathroom – finally! I slowly got down from the bed and walked back to the ward area where I made a dash for the currently empty toilet cubicle. It did cross my mind that maybe I should have remained lying down for half an hour or so, but the nurses reassured me that it would make no difference whatsoever – the uterus was tilted inside the body for a start, and thinking that the embryos might fall out was just plain daft!

I was in the bathroom for some time, unsurprisingly. When I eventually came out Anna was waiting for me. It was nearly 4.45 p.m. and I was conscious that I had to get back to the acupuncture clinic for my after transfer treatment. I slowly dressed whilst the nurse advised me on what I had to do over the next two weeks – similar to on the previous attempts. Six hours after the transfer, around 10.30 p.m., I had to use another Voltarol suppository. Then, twice a day until the pregnancy test, I had to take the progesterone supplement pessary, Cyclogest. I also had to take something called Progynova, an oestrogen hormone replacement, three times a day also until the pregnancy test. It wasn't too much to remember and I was given a sheet with everything listed and when to take it. I thanked the nurses and doctors, who all said they hoped to see me in two weeks for some good news, then we made our way to the car whilst I called the acupuncture clinic to advise them I was on my way. The very pleasant receptionist told me not to worry, just to get there when I could and Daniel would be waiting. I thought again about how understanding and accommodating everyone involved in the process had been this time – private treatment really was so completely different, and I was so grateful to all concerned for that.

We pulled up outside the clinic in Harley Street and I made my way up the steps for the last time. Anna said she'd wait in the car this time as I'd only be half an hour anyway. I realised that I should call my mum really as we'd arranged for her to be at home in Oxford when I returned. As we were running late and she was due to arrive at 6 p.m., I had to let her know. Anna said not to worry, she'd call her and tell her we'd be late. I disappeared through the imposing double doors and popped my head round the reception door to let someone know I'd arrived. The receptionist told me to go straight upstairs where Daniel was waiting for me. Hmm, stairs. I contemplated if it was OK to be climbing stairs so soon then immediately scolded myself. Paranoid, that's what I was.

I smiled and made my way up to the treatment room. Daniel asked me if the transfer had gone alright and how I felt, so I said that despite a tense time of things with the whole bladder episode I was actually incredibly positive. He nodded his approval and began to insert the acupuncture needles. The room was so peaceful, the sun shone outside and I was temporarily in an oasis of tranquillity. I closed my eyes as Daniel left the room, saying he'd be back in twenty minutes. You wouldn't have believed you were in the city; it was so quiet. I decided not to have any soft music playing as I just wanted to be alone with my thoughts, or lack of. I tried to concentrate my mind on absolutely nothing, and it worked.

I awoke a short time later to the sound of the door opening and Daniel returning to remove the needles. When he'd finished I very slowly swung my legs round to the side of the bed – I was really drowsy and must have fallen asleep from the excitement of the day. I thanked Daniel, who told me to make sure I let him know the outcome – he'd had a lot of success with his IVF patients and said he felt really positive about my treatment. I appreciated his interest and said that of course I'd let him know. I paid the receptionist then said a cheery goodbye, opened the front door and walked down the steps to find Anna waiting in the car.

It was rush hour and it would take a while to get home, but it didn't really matter. Anna had managed to get through to my mum so she already knew we'd be quite late. As I sat in the car I felt a bit sore what with all the prodding and pulling but not that much that I couldn't manage – it was OK to take a couple of paracetamol anyway. I looked at Anna and told her that I really fancied a bag of crisps – or two! I hardly ever ate them but I was starting to get really hungry. She laughed then said she'd stop at the first place we saw that would sell them – an off licence or something. It didn't take long before we came across a Boots store, so she pulled up opposite and

I nipped out to buy a few goodies. Traffic was heavy and as I began to rush across the road I suddenly remembered that I really needed to take things easy, so slowed down and took my time.

Once inside I gazed at the shelf – prawn cocktail or salt and vinegar? I couldn't decide so in the end grabbed them both. It wasn't the best nutrition but I'd eaten so carefully for as long as I could remember that the ingestion of a couple of bags of crisps really wasn't going to matter at this point. I looked around to see if there was anything else and my eyes spied Sweet and Sour Pot Noodle. Whilst I couldn't have it until I got home the thought of a Pot Noodle sandwich was just too tempting to resist. I put everything in the basket, quickly paid, and made my way back to the car. I shut the door then turned and grinned at Anna. She wondered what on earth was wrong with me until I pulled the Pot Noodle out of the bag and then she just laughed – she was already familiar with my sandwich obsession!

It took ages to get out of London – the traffic was horrendous. We had to stop at the petrol station on the way to get more fuel too, which was a good job really as I needed the bathroom again. Luckily there was a McDonald's next door so I rather cheekily nipped in there whilst Anna filled the car up. I realised that I hadn't contacted James to let him know it had all gone OK and that we were on our way home, so I quickly dialled his number and left a message. He wouldn't be back until late that night as he had a client meeting early evening, which was one of the reasons why my mum had said she'd drive over for the night.

Back in the car we chatted about the day's events. The traffic had thinned out a little once we were on the M40 and we hoped to be back in Oxford by around 7.45 p.m. We finally reached the outskirts of the city and pulled up in the car park at 8 p.m. My mum was there waiting, sat in her car reading her book. She rushed over as soon as she saw us, asking me how I was and saying that she'd been getting worried as we were taking so long. I thanked Anna for giving up her day to take me and for staying with me during the transfer. I couldn't thank her enough to be honest – there was no way I'd have managed to do the whole day on my own. After seeing us safely in the apartment she left us alone, promising my mum that she'd check in on me over the next few days.

My mum told me to relax whilst she made a cup of tea, then we chatted about what had happened during the day. She wanted to know everything in great detail – even what I'd eaten for lunch. I was tired, but I wasn't able to sleep just yet – I had to wait until 10.30 p.m. so I could take the hormones. I switched the TV on for a while and caught up with the news and what was going on in the world. As soon as I was able I went to bed, exhausted from the day and grateful for knowing that as soon as my head hit the pillow I'd be asleep.

Wednesday, 24th May 2006

My mum woke me up with a cup of tea. James had already disappeared off for the day, so I must have been incredibly tired as he didn't even disturb me as he got ready for work. I sipped my tea and thought about getting up and taking a shower. It was around 9.30 a.m. when the telephone rang – it was the clinic. They said the day before they'd leave the remaining blastocysts another day before checking whether there were any worth freezing, so they were calling to give me an update. Unfortunately the nurse told me that although they were OK they weren't of a good enough quality to survive the freeze and a subsequent thaw.

Whilst it wasn't the best news I found that it didn't upset me. I'd had a feeling that we wouldn't have any to freeze, and we still had one from the second Oxford cycle in cryopreservation anyway, so I wasn't too disappointed. What it did do though was allow me to concentrate on the two embryos I had 'on board'. I was counting on the skill of UCH, along with my body, to make this cycle work. I also knew that I needed to keep busy to prevent my mind from making me crazier than I already was, so I'd decided to go in to work the following week.

In the meantime I was going to take it really easy as I knew I needed to let my body rest properly. I didn't want to just sit down all day though, so after lunch my mum and I walked over to Sainsbury's to pick up something for dinner that night. It wasn't too far and I wasn't in pain, and I definitely needed the fresh air. My mum was staying until Thursday afternoon to make sure I was alright, and it was nice that someone else could sort dinner out for a change – cooking was definitely not one of James's strong points!

Thursday, 25th May 2006

I had a doctor's appointment in Oxford today to collect my sick note for work. My mum drove me down to the surgery then we stopped off at the DVD rental shop on the way back. I needed something to keep me occupied after she'd gone home and until James came back from work. I really wasn't in the mood for reading; I'd done so much of that recently, both online and in books, and I'd temporarily got a bit fed up with it. A funny movie to divert my attention for a few hours so that I didn't have to think was perfect.

After a sandwich lunch my mum left at around 1.30 p.m. We said goodbye, with her promising to call me later that evening to see how I was, then she set off for home. I walked back up the stairs to the apartment and closed the door behind me. I was on my own again. I thought I might struggle to be alone; to keep the thoughts in my head from overtaking everything else, but I actually felt quite peaceful. There were thirteen days to go until the pregnancy test, and it was the last time I'd put myself through two weeks of limbo. Whilst I knew that on testing day my heart would be in my mouth, I also knew that it would be the start of a new life, one way or the other. I just had to get through two weeks of constant analysis – every single twinge, ache, and stomach rumble would, I knew, come under such scrutiny that my head would attach meaning to absolutely everything. I had to force myself to focus on remaining in my current state of calm optimism.

Tuesday, 30th May 2006

I went back to work this morning and I was glad of the distraction. I'd had cramp-like pain all day. It hadn't worked.

Wednesday, 31st May 2006

I noticed a small amount of discharge. My insides felt hollow. I couldn't handle this – it was too much.

Monday, 5ᵗʰ June 2006

After two days of symptoms, I'd had three days of none, followed by pain all Sunday night. Not strong, really worrying pain, but still pain nonetheless. I'd somehow managed to get through the past five days without going completely mad, although I'd been on edge the whole time. I'd fluctuated between complete depression and sadness to extreme positivity that I'd got this far again. During the last cycle I'd experienced discharge on day eleven and the result had been negative. It was day eleven of this cycle, and with two days to go until I could test, the apprehension was unbearable.

Wednesday, 7ᵗʰ June 2006

The big day had arrived. It was also 5 o'clock in the morning and I was wide awake. Part of me wanted to know, part of me just wanted to bury my head in the sand. Irrational had become my second name recently, and there I was, about to find out which direction my life was about to take, with a sudden urge to just make it all go away. I stared at the ceiling, trying to decide if testing a couple of hours early would alter the outcome. I told you I'd become irrational.

James was still half asleep but I nudged him anyway and asked him what he thought. He said he didn't mind. A typical male response then, and really unhelpful. I sighed and hauled myself out of bed. I hadn't noticed any further discharge since last Wednesday, and whilst I was still experiencing a little pain it wasn't the type of intense cramping that would come with a period. How desperately I hoped it had worked – there was only one way to find out.

I sauntered over to the bathroom and took a couple of First Response pregnancy test sticks out of the cupboard.

I'd bought three packets, just in case. There was no way you could rely on one, and if, just IF, it was positive I'd have to do another couple of tests just to make sure.

I sat down and unwrapped the packet. I could hear and feel my heart beating in my chest. This was it, moment of truth. In a few minutes I'd know. I opened the toilet lid and held the test stick mid-stream, making sure it was wet enough for an accurate result. I put the protective cap on the end of the stick then washed my hands. The anticipation was killing me already, and I had to wait another agonising three minutes.

Or so I thought. I turned round to dry my hands when I glanced at the test stick sitting there on the windowsill. Staring at me, quite clearly, were two bright pink lines. Really bright pink lines. Two of them. Two bright pink lines. Oh. My. God. It had been what, thirty seconds, and there it was, staring me in the face – *two bright pink lines*. I had to sit down again. I was completely overwhelmed. My insides were all over the place and I just sat there and laughed. And cried. And laughed some more. I couldn't believe it. I just couldn't believe it. Two pink lines, straight away. Wow. That was a definite positive result. I was pregnant. I couldn't believe that I was actually saying that I WAS PREGNANT! My brain wouldn't function. I didn't know what to do and I just sat there in a state of disbelief. I had to tell James – oh, I'd forgotten about James. I'd forgotten about absolutely everything else in the world. I was in the moment and I wanted it to last forever. I pulled myself together sufficiently enough to walk over to his side of the bed then prodded him. "It's worked," I said. "James, I'm pregnant." He opened his eyes and smiled.

Chapter 9

Bump!

It was still only 5.30 a.m. I couldn't possibly call my mum at that time in the morning, could I? I decided to wait another half an hour. I knew she'd already be awake but somehow it didn't seem right to ring her at that time. I lay back on the bed and a huge wave of relief came from nowhere. Tears began to fall but this time a huge smile accompanied them. I was in a moment of disbelief and everything felt upside down and unsettled but exciting at the same time. Was this what people meant when they described elation? All those emotions from the past couple of years came right back and they were so overpowering. I had to get up to try and distract myself and calm down.

I checked the clock; five minutes to six. I couldn't wait any longer – I had to call my mum. I went into the living room, picked up the phone and dialled the number. It felt like ages but it must only have been a couple of seconds until I heard my mum on the other end. I didn't even say hello. I just blurted out, "It's positive!"

I heard a sharp intake of breath, quickly followed by laughter. She was absolutely ecstatic. She asked me how I felt and I tried to describe the sense of disbelief, without much success. We chatted for a while longer until she had to get ready to go to work, then I said I'd call her later once

I knew what the clinic wanted me to do. By the time I'd eaten as much breakfast as I could stomach due to all the excitement, it was getting on for 7.45 a.m. I had to call the clinic and hoped that someone would be there so early.

I dialled the number and the receptionist picked up straight away. I asked her if there was anyone I could speak to about my pregnancy test, and luckily one of the nurses was available. I explained that I'd done the pregnancy test a couple of hours ago and that the result had been an immediate positive. The first thing the nurse said was, "Congratulations!" I laughed and thanked her, then she asked me if I could get in to the clinic that day so that they could confirm it by doing a blood test. I said I could and arranged to be there for 2.30 p.m. I put the phone down then quickly got myself dressed. I decided to go into work anyway – I could stay until lunchtime then catch the 1 p.m. train.

I gathered my things and made sure I had my book with me for the train journey, although I probably wouldn't be able to concentrate long enough to read any of it, then I made my way downstairs to my car. I don't know how I did it but one minute I was in the car park at home and the next minute I was in the one at work. I'd driven on auto-pilot and couldn't even remember the journey. To say I was excited was a huge understatement and I think I was still in a state of disbelief. The blood test would help in that respect – the hormone, hCG, would only be present if the embryo had implanted into the uterus, indicating pregnancy. It was the same hormone they'd tested for at Oxford after the first ICSI cycle, when the initial result had been borderline and I'd miscarried.

I rummaged in my bag for my security card then made my way up the stairs to the first floor. I pushed open the lobby door then the office one and saw Ali look up straight away, seemingly surprised to see me. I didn't wait for her to ask – I just said "Hi," then sat down and said, "It's positive." She beamed at me and gave me a big hug, saying it was fantastic news. She was so happy that at last it had worked for us.

I told her that I had to be in London for a 2.30 p.m. clinic appointment so would have to leave a bit earlier than usual, although I'd be back in the following day as there was no need to have any more time off. Ali made us both a cup of tea and I tried to get on with my work, although I don't know how I managed to finish it as I was in a complete daze all morning. My eyes kept watching the clock slowly ticking by, until eventually it was time to leave to get to the station.

I sat on the train looking at the pages in my book but paying absolutely no attention to them whatsoever. Was I really pregnant? I didn't feel it, but then what was I supposed to feel? All the signs I'd been willing myself to have to indicate pregnancy had not materialised at all. Now, the nearer I came to the clinic and the 'true' test of pregnancy i.e. the blood test, the more nervous I became. What if the test sticks had been faulty?

My irrational thoughts were interrupted by the tannoy announcement saying we'd shortly be arriving at Padding-ton station. I snapped out of my self-indulgent thinking and got my things together. It was quite warm today and I only had to carry my bag and a lightweight jacket. I made my way out through the concourse and towards the taxi rank. There wasn't a queue so I immediately jumped in the nearest cab and set off for the clinic.

When I arrived the waiting room was only half full. I confirmed my appointment with reception and was immediately sent downstairs to the procedure area where the blood tests were done. I sat down on one of the waiting area chairs and stared at the various pictures of magnified embryos displayed on the wall in front of me. I thought about those two pink lines I'd seen that morning and it felt weird, almost as if it wasn't quite real just yet. I needed to know exactly what my hormone level was before I'd truly be able to accept it.

After a few minutes and a quick flick through the magazines, a nurse popped her head around the door and called me through to one of the vacant office cubicles. She smiled and congratulated me, then explained that she'd take a couple of blood samples so that they could confirm the pregnancy. I'd find out later that day too; they would give me a call to let me know the result as soon as it came through from the lab. I rolled up my sleeve and waited for the all too familiar needle. It took a couple of moments before she could find a vein that would do the job – as I'd been jabbed that often all the good ones had been rendered pretty useless by now. After the vials were full and as I made my way back up the stairs the nurse's words echoed in my head; I'd get a call later on that day to let me know the result. Another couple of hours of being on tenterhooks loomed.

I exited the clinic via the back entrance and walked underneath the archway and onto Grey's Inn Road. I suddenly realised that I was absolutely exhausted. The events of the day had completely drained me and I felt that familiar desire to get home again. There was no way I wanted to walk all the way back down Oxford Street. There'd be far too many people and I longed to be on my own so that I could just 'be', knowing that I no longer had to think about treatments, or drugs, or appointments.

I walked up to King's Cross and hailed a taxi to Paddington. Once at the station, I walked through the concourse to the departures screens and saw that a train to Didcot was due to leave ten minutes later. After a quick visit to Starbucks for my chai tea latte fix, I made my way to the platform with a few minutes to spare. As the train slowly moved away from the station I looked at my watch – it was quarter to four. In a few hours' time the events of the past few years would come to an end. Whilst the pregnancy test had been positive that morning I still needed the comfort of knowing for sure, which hopefully the blood test could provide. It would take just one phone call to confirm that that period of my life was over and I'd be able to start looking forward to an exciting new one.

Once back at home I put the kettle on for a cup of tea then flopped down on the sofa. No coffee for me for nine months – it seemed that no sooner had one set of paranoid thinking ended, than another began!

Just before 6 p.m. and as I was about to change the TV channel to catch up on the news the telephone rang. I nervously lifted the receiver to be greeted by a nurse from the clinic. It was the result of the blood test. I held my breath for a couple of moments then heard her voice say that the good news was that I was definitely pregnant, and the even better news was that my level of beta hCG hormone was 2,758. She said that it was a very high reading and at this point it was excellent news.

There was no doubt about it, I was most definitely pregnant! To say I was beside myself was an understatement for sure. I could feel the tears pricking the back of my eyes again and my face must have displayed one huge beaming grin. It was all just so unbelievable, even after absolute proof. I made myself concentrate long enough to hear the rest of the conversation as she went on to say something about going back for a second blood test to check hCG levels in about a week's time. She explained that in a healthy pregnancy the hormone should double every two to three days, so we agreed that I'd go back to the clinic the following Tuesday for another test.

I thanked the nurse for calling then replaced the receiver, walked over to the window and stared out at the gardens below. It was all so unreal and the feeling was intense. My emotions were all over the place and I had to take a few minutes to try and centre myself, although I struggled to control what was a complete surge of happiness. I had to find a balance; a way of dealing with my powerful feelings, or I'd be a wreck by the end of the weekend. I thought about my mum and how thrilled she'd be, then picked up the phone again and dialled her number. I had to tell her that she was very definitely going to be a grandma!

Tuesday, 13ᵗʰ June 2006

hCG level, 14,852. Perfect, apparently, meaning no more blood tests. The next hurdle? The first scan, due in just over one week's time. All I had to do was sit back and enjoy every minute of being pregnant.

Saturday, 17th June 2006

I'd already started to worry about the impending scan scheduled for the following week. What if it didn't show anything? What if it all wasn't real? All these thoughts were completely irrational, but unfortunately for me no matter how hard I tried to dispel them with positive and non-emotional thinking they just didn't go away. Everyone must have thought I was crazy; I'd just had a positive pregnancy test for goodness sake, why wasn't I able to just be happy and accept it?

I can't describe why I felt like I did, I just did. It was so precious that I suppose I needed someone to tell me with absolute certainty that nine months later I'd give birth to a healthy baby. I was convinced that it being the last opportunity in my life had something to do with it; made it all the more crucial. I tried to ignore such negative thinking as much as I could but it was always there, in the back of my mind. Not usually one for wishing a life away, I did, however, just want to get to the following Thursday when I would, hopefully, see the evidence with my own eyes. Surely that would be enough?

Thursday, 22nd June 2006

It was four weeks since the embryos had been transferred and two weeks since the positive pregnancy test. The past week or so had, unexpectedly, been quite tough. I'd assumed, probably naïvely that all the anxiety would just disappear overnight. Whether it was just a part of my character or whether it was completely normal to feel the way I did was irrelevant. The fact was that my dream world of everything being absolutely perfect had lasted for approximately four days, from the previous Tuesday to the Saturday.

Last night, however, I'd been surprisingly more settled. Although still slightly agitated, I'd managed to still the inner voices sufficiently to realise that whatever we saw on the scan the following day there was not a thing I could do about it. My hormone levels had been where they should have been, if not higher than expected, and I felt physically fine. In fact I found myself in a state of excited apprehension – it was going to be an interesting day.

I was due at the clinic at 12 noon. James had gone into work early as usual and I'd arranged to have the day off. It was my last appointment at the clinic, after which I'd transfer to my local hospital and the midwife for the rest of my pregnancy, as normal. No more faffing about with trains and taxis, although to be honest I'd actually quite enjoyed going into London for treatment – it had definitely been the right decision.

I was meeting James at his office and as it was a decent enough day weather-wise I decided to walk; I had to make sure I got enough gentle exercise anyway. I made my way to Sussex Place then walked through Hyde Park Gardens via the Mews. From there it was a short distance to Marble Arch then across to Berkeley Square, past the American Embassy. I'd become so used to the route over the years I could do it with my eyes closed. Once I was there the receptionist phoned James to tell him I'd arrived then we waited on the pavement outside the office for a cab; it usually took only a couple of minutes before one turned up.

The taxi weaved its way in and out of the traffic and we chatted about what we we'd hopefully see on the ultrasound, and admitted that we were both very nervous, but also incredibly excited. It was another one of those once in a lifetime moments that we would never get to experience again. I wish there was some way I could have captured it all rather than have to rely on memory.

As we approached the clinic I felt the nerves and apprehension start to kick in again. James paid the driver whilst I made my way to reception, then we sat down in the fairly empty waiting area. I picked up a magazine and began to read one of the articles when a doctor appeared and called my name. I looked at James as I stood up and let out a huge sigh. Of all the cliff-hanger moments to date, this was by far the worst in terms of the anticipation. I felt my heart pounding in my chest – what if the doctor couldn't see anything on the monitor?

We were led into the now familiar small ultrasound room. I sat on the bed whilst James found a chair and pulled it up next to me so he could see the monitor, then the doctor began by introducing himself. He said his name was Mr Ertan Saridogan and that he'd be doing the ultrasound scan to confirm the presence of an embryo and check that it had implanted in my uterus and not the fallopian tubes. I knew it was procedure and everything but I just wanted him to get on with it for goodness sake; I really had to bite my tongue to stop me from blurting it out! The suspense surely wasn't good for my mental health either, not to mention that I had to have yet another full bladder. I removed my lower clothes then lay down on the bed with the cover over myself to protect my modesty. I chuckled to myself at that point. Any modesty I'd had in the first place was long gone by now.

Mr Saradogan left the room whilst I made myself comfortable, then thirty seconds or so later he returned, smiled, and asked if we were ready. I looked at James then nodded, took a deep breath and said a rather mousy, "Yes." Mr Saradogan turned the screen towards us and began to view the images. After repeatedly moving the transducer to show various angles he started to explain what he could see on the screen. I held my breath for a second then heard him say, "This dark shape here is the uterine cavity, and," pointing to the circular shape inside it, "this is the yolk sac, and next to it is your embryo." He continued to tell us that the slight flicker we were seeing coming from the embryo was its heartbeat. I opened my mouth but nothing came out. I was completely speechless. I just didn't know what to say or do – I think it's called dumbstruck. The only thing I could manage was a huge grin from ear to ear that gave me the appearance of being a complete nutter. My insides flipped over and over again; the feeling was just overwhelming. It was real, completely, one hundred per cent, without a doubt, real!

Mr Saradogan gave us his congratulations then, after a couple more clicks of the mouse, told us that given the size and measurements our estimated due date was 8th February 2007. He carried on checking the rest of my uterine area to make sure everything all looked OK before I could get dressed, and was just about to remove the probe when he said, "Hold on a minute, what's this?" I looked at James in a panic then quickly back at the doctor again. "Aha," he said, "and here I can see another embryo, with an equally strong heartbeat." Well, my jaw just dropped as I looked at James once more. It was twins.

I didn't know whether to laugh or cry, it was way beyond anything I'd ever imagined or hoped for. Bloody hell. Twins. No way. My mum would have a heart attack when I told her! Unless James beat her to it – I looked at him again and saw that he'd gone as white as a sheet. I didn't know whether it was from shock or what, but at least he was smiling as well. I felt like I was floating on air and everything around me melted into a time-stopping fuzzy haze. I was in my own little bubble of a perfect world. Mr Saradogan switched off the monitor and replaced the probe in its holder, then finished off by explaining that as each embryo was in its own sac, the likelihood was that both of them had implanted successfully.

Just wow. I had difficulty letting it all sink in. Feeling like jelly I didn't know if my legs would work properly once I got off the bed but work they did, and a good job too – if I was having twins I'd need to get as much gentle exercise as I could for as long as possible. Oh no, I was going to look like a brick outhouse wasn't I? I laughed to myself – how unbelievably exciting – I'd always wanted twins, and after everything we'd been through it was just amazing. I looked at James again and said, "It's twins." He grinned and replied, "I know, I'm seeing pound signs in front of my eyes." I laughed again. That was so true, and coupled with the total cost of about £15,000 for the three cycles we'd probably be in debt for the rest of our lives but, irresponsibly, I just didn't care.

James checked that I was happy to get back to the station on my own then said a quick goodbye as he had a client meeting he had to rush to. I continued walking towards Chancery Lane tube station, took a right turn into

Bloomsbury Way, then carried on to Oxford Street. It was only a couple of miles and it gave me the chance to be alone and contemplate the fantastic news. I think I must have walked all the way with a massive smile plastered across my face. The fact that I had two little people inside was still very difficult to get my head around even though I'd just seen it with my own eyes. I wanted to tell my mum and dad, but I also sort of wanted to keep it to myself for a little while. I decided to have one precious half an hour when it was just me and my thoughts. It's difficult to explain but it felt as though being alone allowed me to acknowledge all the built up emotion from the past few years.

I finally arrived at Oxford Circus and, with the aim of calling my parents, turned into a side street to try and avoid the noise. I nervously dialled their number and waited. It rang. And rang. And rang. Unbelievable – nobody was in! Either that or they were in the garden and couldn't hear the phone. I sighed and wondered what to do next. I'd have to keep trying periodically so didn't really want to wander too far, and I was definitely hungry so I had to fix that for sure. I glanced down Oxford Street and spied John Lewis just up the road on the right-hand side. Ah, perfect. I'd have a sandwich or something and a cup of tea. I wandered in to the store and took the escalator up to the fifth floor to the main restaurant, The Place To Eat.

There was a wide choice available including salads, omelettes, chef cooked main meals, crepes and patisserie. I thought for a moment – I really fancied an omelette but wasn't sure if that was safe to eat. Was it advisable for a pregnant woman to eat eggs? It suddenly dawned on me that I was about to embark upon a whole new completely unexpected experience. Such a simple thing as what to eat had turned into a minefield of can I or can't I? Was I just a tiny bit paranoid? Other people seemed to do just fine in pregnancy without resorting to analysing everything, but then I wasn't in the position of most people when they were pregnant.

I didn't realise it at the time but after what I'd endured to get to this stage, the absolute pricelessness of what was inside me would take over every single thought and action for the next nine months. There wasn't a thing I was able to do about it; for me it felt completely normal to question such small things. I thought for a second then decided it was probably OK to have an omelette as long as it was cooked properly but to be on the safe side I'd just stick to a sandwich instead. I made my way over to the salad and sandwich section to see what was available. First up, prawns. Er, no, definitely not. Salmon and dill? Nope, that wasn't wise either. Goat cheese? Hmm. Was that considered a soft cheese? Better not, just in case. This was getting ridiculous now. I took another look – the only options left were roast turkey or houmous and roasted vegetables. That'd do, I'd have the houmous. You couldn't go wrong with beans and vegetables – no danger there. I took the plate and put it on my tray. At least it was easier deciding what to drink; no coffee, no alcohol, just tea or water, so I chose both.

I paid for my meal then scanned the room for a vacant table. It was just after the lunchtime rush so I managed to find one fairly easily, next to the window. I slowly ate my meal, all the time feeling like I was in a daze. Our lives would change dramatically. I'd dreamed about the idea of having twins all my life, ever since my mum had been to see a clairvoyant when I was a child who told her that either me or my brother would do so. I was sure it was just coincidence but it had always stuck in my mind. Once I knew we'd have to have treatment I'd always hoped that it would be possible but to find out it was going to be real was beyond words.

I finished my sandwich and checked my watch. I really had to try and call my parents again. I got my things together and made my way over towards the escalator, glancing at the store directory as I walked past, stopping in my tracks. Apparently I was only one floor away from the nursery department and I had to pass through it on my way down. I thought for a moment then berated myself for being so daft – I'd only got confirmation a couple of hours ago for goodness sake, I couldn't possibly start looking at equipment already. Could I?

Excitement got the better of me – the temptation was just too much. I reached the bottom of the escalator and casually walked over to the nursery section. Luckily it was quite busy so I wasn't immediately jumped on by a sales assistant. I think I would have just giggled if someone had approached me. I took a look around and couldn't believe how much stuff there was. This baby lark definitely had the potential to get completely out of hand. Was it all really that necessary? I could see that I'd have to start implementing a bit of restraint!

I spied the display with the prams and pushchairs and started searching for a double buggy. This was just too ridiculous; I was having real difficulty taking anything seriously. I took a quick look at the models they had on the stand then made myself scarce before I could be accosted by a well-meaning salesperson.

Back down on the ground floor and with a recovered composure, I wondered where I could go that would be quiet enough for my mum to hear me on my mobile. There was a street running parallel to the store that looked fairly promising so I exited the side doors to have a look. It was quiet enough. I turned and wandered down the street a bit further to make sure there was sufficient distance between me and the Oxford Street traffic. As I nervously dialled my mum and dad's number again I looked at the large window display, coincidentally filled with items from the baby and nursery section, including twin buggies. That gave me an idea.

I waited a couple of moments for my mum to pick up the phone – surely she'd answer this time. It wasn't long before I heard a click and my mum's voice on the end of the line. I told her I'd had the scan, everything was as it should be and that there was no question about it, she was definitely going to be a grandma. She was really happy for us and so glad that it all looked OK. I thought for a moment then nonchalantly said, "I know it's a bit soon but I'm just looking at prams in the window at John Lewis." She laughed and agreed that maybe it was a little bit early to be looking for equipment already. I carried on, "I particularly like the double buggies…it's twins."

I heard a sharp intake of breath then, "Oh Tru, that's wonderful. What fantastic news!" I knew my mum was beside herself; I could tell by the tone in her voice. In fact she probably cried for an hour once she put the phone down. She said, "Hold on a minute, let me put your dad on. Just tell him what you told me." So I did, all over again. My dad sounded really excited too, although at least he managed to keep it together slightly better than my mum!

We chatted for a few minutes more then I had to go and catch the train before it got too late. I said I'd ring her later on when I got home, although before I disconnected the call I adamantly reminded her to Not. Tell. Anybody! On the one hand I was itching to tell the whole world but on the other, if anything went wrong I would be devastated and wouldn't be able to deal with friends and relatives knowing. We'd discussed what to do about telling people as soon as I'd had the positive pregnancy test – we wanted to wait until the twelve week scan, although it was going to be very hard keeping it a secret for so long.

Saturday, 24th June 2006

I just couldn't help myself, could I? All that time during treatment going in to bookstores and completely avoiding the pregnancy and parenting section irrationally thinking I might jeopardise my chances, so what did I do at the first opportunity in a bookstore? Exactly. Bought a book about twins and pregnancy! It did, however take me an absolute age to make a decision as to which one – there was so much choice. Most of them consisted of advice on what to do and what not to do, often with conflicting information depending on whose opinion it was. It was too overwhelming, and I did consider just not bothering at all. I knew that I'd probably read a couple and disagree with what they said anyway. What I needed was a book about facts, not a how-to manual. In the end I decided to go for a twin specific option – *Twins! Pregnancy, Birth and the First Year of Life*[iii]. It covered everything from prenatal care, a monthly summary of growth stages by week, then delivery and birth up to the first birthday. Along with a few pregnancy magazines that would be enough anyway; as I'd already found out, sometimes too much information was counter-productive.

I paid for the book whilst James bought the newspapers then, after picking up a couple of magazines, we made ourselves comfortable in the coffee shop. We talked about where we'd been that morning – after finding out about the twins on Thursday then coming back home to the apartment we realised that we'd have to reconsider our living arrangements.

Our apartment was on the first floor which would have been manageable with one baby, but having two changed everything. Simple logistics such as getting both babies up the stairs at the same time would be impossible. No-one was allowed to leave anything in the lobby either so whilst we may have been able to persuade the other residents to accept a small pushchair, parking a double buggy underneath the stairs would definitely not be an option. Being my usual resourceful self, once I'd got back from work on the Friday I scoured the websites of local estate agents and found a couple of possibilities that suited us in terms of location and appropriate size. One of them was available to view the following morning, so I'd made an appointment for 11 a.m.

The house was in a small village called Sutton Courtenay, near Abingdon in Oxfordshire. At the time we lived on the outskirts of Oxford, and as the village was twelve miles away from our current location it would be quite a change not being able to just pop into the city. However, it would be much more convenient for James to get to London as the main train line passed through Didcot, and it would be about three and a half miles from the station to the house. Although we could afford to wait a little while longer before we moved we did need to find a property that ticked all the boxes – enough bedrooms for everybody plus visitors, enough space for a home office, and adequate parking for two cars. Not to mention all the paraphernalia that we needed such as two of everything and the ability to get a double buggy through the front door!

The house was located in a small, gated community, and was laid out over three floors. The top floor was in the eaves and would be perfect for an office area. Outside there was a front and rear garden and a double garage with a driveway. We considered our options and came to the conclusion that we didn't actually have any. There was certainly nothing suitable in Oxford itself and as we had to give one month's notice on our current apartment, and I really wanted to be moved and settled before I started to resemble an elephant, we called the estate agent and confirmed that we'd take it.

Sunday, 2nd July 2006

It had been a fairly uneventful week for once. I was grateful for that, as things had happened so fast recently that my head needed time to assimilate it all. The thought of the chaos of twins hadn't even hit me yet; I'd just been living in a bubble for the whole week. I'd been trying to do things as normally as I had prior to being pregnant, although every time I did something I found myself questioning whether it was right. For instance, I knew that I had to make sure I got enough exercise, especially so with it being twins, but on the other hand I was slightly afraid of overdoing things to the point where it could be detrimental. I still had my gym membership and although I wasn't going to run at eight miles an hour on the treadmill I had to do something. I took advantage of the reclining bicycle machine, although it was incredibly boring and I hated cycling anyway, but at least it kept the circulation going.

As far as the new house went, we'd already asked my parents if they'd like to see it so they drove down on Saturday night ready for viewing it on Sunday morning. It was important to me that they liked it, and after getting their subsequent approval we headed into Oxford for lunch. There was a really nice restaurant in the High Street called Quod that was part of the Old Bank Hotel. We'd been before several times and it was always a good option for Sunday lunch.

By the time we'd finished it was getting on for 3 o'clock so we went back to our apartment for a cup of tea before my parents started their journey back home. My mum found it really hard to leave. I knew that she really wanted to be around for me and was sorry that we lived so far away. I was too to be honest. Although Anna wasn't far away and I saw her quite often, there really was no substitute for family being around, especially your mum. I felt that she'd miss out on being a part of it and it was such a shame for both of us. Still, it was very early days and there'd be plenty of time for me to travel up to see her and my dad. I also knew it wouldn't be long before they'd be back.

Wednesday, 5th July 2006
Nine weeks pregnant. I'd been to work as normal since the beginning of the week and today was just another one of those days. I finished at 1 p.m. then went straight home.

I hadn't been on the Fertility Friends website for a while so thought I'd log in and catch up on some of the threads. It was tempting to look at the section for multiples, but I was in two minds as to whether it would be a good thing or not. I scanned the forum list and saw that there was a section just for pregnancy and then a section in the parenting bit for twins, triplets or more. I thought for a moment then clicked on the standard pregnancy threads. Did I really want to know so far in advance about how difficult life was with twin babies – er, no. I decided that the simple pregnancy forum would be more relevant at the moment, and there was sure to be a thread or two about multiple pregnancies anyway.

I spent the next couple of hours just reading other people's posts, then when I got bored of that began on the pregnancy websites. I realised that I'd have to keep it in check though – you could spend the whole week just whiling away time on various information sites, and they all said the same things really. I glanced at my watch and realised it was nearly 6 p.m. James would be home soon but I was quite hungry already and decided to have dinner a little earlier. I found that I was quite ravenous just lately and put it down to the demands of growing two little people.

After a very tasty mushroom risotto I cleared the pots into the dishwasher then flicked the kettle on whilst I went to the bathroom. That was another thing – I seemed to have a bladder the size of a pea these days – that had better improve after the twins arrived. I checked the bathroom tissue just before flushing, which had become a bit of habit after three rounds of IVF, and saw what was, quite obviously, a large, red stain. Oh God. I was bleeding.

Anxiously I sat down again. I could feel my heart beating in my chest and I had that horrible knot of stress in my stomach. How could I be bleeding? It wasn't from implantation, I was nine weeks pregnant. I tried to hold the tears back and not panic. James wasn't home yet but I had to tell someone so I called my mum, in spite of her being a hundred and twenty miles away. I didn't want to worry her but I couldn't cope with it on my own. I went into the bedroom, sat on the edge of the bed then picked up the phone, and with shaking hands dialled her mobile number. She probably wouldn't pick up as it was only just after 6.30 p.m. and she usually went to my grandma's house after work before going home.

I waited for the tone and after a couple of rings she answered. As soon as I heard her voice I broke down. I couldn't keep the tears from falling; I was absolutely desperate. In between sobs I told her that I was bleeding and that I thought I was losing the babies. I heard her voice wobble as she spoke but she managed to keep it together as she told me to sit tight and wait for James to come home, then we could go straight to A&E. She tried to encourage me by saying that the bleeding might not even mean anything, and although I tried to believe it and in my heart I willed it to be so, my head just wouldn't stop running off on its own, imagining the worst.

As we spoke I heard the sound of James's key in the front door. I quickly told my mum that I'd call her later then replaced the receiver and rushed to the kitchen. James could see from my tear-stained face that I was distressed and he looked worried as he asked me what was wrong. Needless to say, as soon as I'd managed to blurt out what had happened I found myself being frogmarched down the apartment stairs and into the car. I was still in a bit of a state but the action of actually doing something gave me a reason to focus and I managed to stop sobbing sometime during the journey to the hospital.

James dropped me off whilst he found a parking space and I made my way through to the A&E reception area. It wasn't busy and I was able to speak to someone straight away. The lady behind the desk took all my details and asked me what the problem was, then I was asked to take a seat and wait to be called. James arrived in the meantime, and we both just sat there in silence. Although I'd managed to stem the flow of tears, inside I felt wretched and I was sick to my stomach with worry.

At ten minutes to eight we were taken through to the triage area where we were greeted by the same doctor who saw us the last time I'd been to A&E with that panic attack. She remembered us too, and was very understanding. As she took my blood pressure, a normal 118/78, she asked me what had happened. I told her that I'd been bleeding since late that afternoon and that it had contained some clots, although I didn't have any cramp-like pain. The doctor then explained that the first thing she had to do was check to see if my cervix was open or closed. Teamed with the bleeding, even though it was a small amount, if it was open it would more than likely indicate an impending miscarriage[iv]. If it was closed and the 'plug' was still intact then it wasn't such bad news and it would take further investigations to work out why I was bleeding.

I let out a huge sigh and fought very hard to remain neutral until we found out what was going on. Externally

I probably came across as being very together. Internally I was in torment. My stomach was in a knot once more and I had an aching pain in the back of my neck that gave me an almighty headache. I was conscious that the obvious stress wouldn't be doing me any good either but I was just unable to control it.

A nurse appeared at the side of the cubicle pushing a wheelchair. I had to see a gynaecologist in the women's department so was transferred to the ward to be examined. I wasn't being checked in as a patient just yet though – they'd wait to see the results of the examination first before deciding if that was necessary. I checked my watch as I was wheeled through the corridors up to the gynaecology ward. It was 8.25 p.m. My mum would be going out of her mind with worry by now – I had to call her as soon as we had any news.

James walked by my side in complete silence. There wasn't really anything to say anyway, we just had to wait until we'd seen the doctor. I'd rather hoped not to be seeing the gynaecology ward again to be honest, what with having stayed there the year before when I'd got OHSS. I knew it would bring back sad memories; something I really didn't need. I tried to banish those thoughts from my mind. It was just geography after all.

We arrived on the ward and I was taken straight in to an examination room. The doctor had been notified that we were on our way up so he was already waiting. He explained that he was going to check the state of my cervix, which would then tell him more about what we could expect to happen next. It wouldn't hurt as all he had to do was shine a very large light inside so he could see. It would just be like having a cervical smear exam – uncomfortable but not painful. I took a few deep breaths then lay down in position on the examination table. James stayed in the room with me and took my hand as the doctor began to prepare the speculum. I could feel my heart pounding in my chest. The unnerving feelings of anticipation seemed to go on forever, and as the speculum was inserted I gazed at the ceiling, then closed my eyes and tried to relax, trying to picture being anywhere but the hospital.

After what felt like an eternity but was probably just a couple of seconds the doctor spoke. My cervix was still closed. The ensuing heavy sigh was inevitable and I was amazed that I managed to keep it together. As I got dressed he explained that whilst my cervix was closed they still needed to know where the bleeding was coming from and what it meant. All they could confirm at that point in time was that I wasn't having a miscarriage. My condition was, however, technically considered a threatened miscarriage and the next step would be an ultrasound scan to see what was going on inside. Given it was late evening that wouldn't happen until the following day at the earliest.

From the hospital's point of view it looked like the emergency was over. From my point of view I didn't understand. Why couldn't they just scan me now? The even worse news was that they were unable to do it until Friday, 7th July, as the gynaecology clinic didn't open on Thursdays. I was completely gobsmacked – why couldn't they scan me in a different department then? Surely they had other ultrasound machines? What about the ones in the hospital's fertility unit? Didn't they understand how stressful it would be to have to wait two days until I could be seen? There was, however, nothing I could do. It wasn't a medical emergency and the impression I got was that as far as they were concerned neither my state of mind nor wellbeing in the meantime were considered a priority. They had to follow procedure, and that classed me as just a number in a waiting list. Reassured that my cervix was still closed, yet deeply worried and unsettled , not knowing whether I'd have a miscarriage at any time, we made our way back to the car and home.

Friday, 7th July 2006

It was 9 a.m. when I parked my car in the hospital car park, ready for my appointment at the gynaecology clinic at 9.30 a.m. The department is located in the Women's Centre at the front of the building near the A&E department, and although I hadn't been to that particular part of the hospital before it wasn't difficult to find. I registered my arrival with the reception desk then sat down to wait. I'd considered taking a book with me as it was pretty much a given that any medical appointment almost never ran on time, but decided there was no point as I wasn't exactly in the mood for reading anyway.

I sat on the front row directly facing the door to the ultrasound room. Every time it opened and a nurse walked out with a clipboard I waited expectantly. After I'd seen two other ladies called into their appointments then leave, it was my turn.

The nurse called my name and I was up like a shot and on the examination table in no time; I was desperate to know what was going on. The nurse began by recounting everything that had happened right up until two nights ago when I'd had the bleed. She was very kind and calm, and as her assistant dimmed the lights to help with viewing the ultrasound screen she squirted the cold jelly medium on to my abdomen. The room went quiet whilst the nurse moved the transducer around to get a full picture. Once again it felt as though my heart had stopped, as I found myself holding my breath for a couple of seconds until I heard her say that both babies were perfectly normal for age and that she couldn't see anything that looked out of the ordinary.

Whilst that was some comfort I wanted to know why I'd had some bleeding, even though I wasn't in any pain. All she could confirm was that she couldn't see a reason why, so at that point she wasn't able to say. She was completely untroubled by it, whereas I was climbing the walls imagining that it was all over. I was in the dark and out of control of absolutely everything and I knew I'd be in a heightened state of agitation until the bleeding stopped.

The nurse suggested that I monitored how things went and that if I was still worried after a few days and the bleeding continued, I should contact them to make another appointment. I just nodded and said OK, then resignedly got off the bed. I felt deflated. Perhaps unrealistically I'd expected to have a definitive answer. All I saw in front of me was a long stretch of waiting to see and I didn't know how to deal with that. Living day to day, not knowing whether I would actually have my babies or not, after everything we'd gone through, would be incredibly tough. I felt stressed and my insides were in knots, which in turn made me feel really guilty as I knew how important it was not to get worked up during pregnancy.

As I left the hospital I contacted James and my mum

to let them both know the outcome. The positive news was that there wasn't any obvious problem that had been identified on the ultrasound, and I told my mum that all I could do was focus on that for the next few days or weeks, or however long it took until the bleeding stopped. Admittedly it had become patchier and it wasn't fresh bright red blood any more, which at least meant there was no imminent problem.

I got in my car, switched the radio on then thought rationally for a minute. I had this problem and I had to deal with it. Nothing I could do would change anything. Either I was going to carry these babies or I wasn't, and I had to try and believe in myself and stay focused as much as possible. Fervent hope was a strange concept for me though, being more inclined towards scientific facts than huge leaps of faith in something intangible. I had to clear my head and trust my body. My gut feelings had deserted me so I didn't even have those as comfort. Although it would be hard I had to try and let go of the disproportionate panic and begin a strategy of acceptance. I sighed, drove out of the car park and made my way to work.

Friday, 14th July 2006
Ten weeks pregnant. I have no idea how I got through the previous weekend. During the week I was at work which helped to take my mind off things, at least for the mornings anyway, and I'd really tried to concentrate on not thinking too much – trying to forget I was pregnant, if you like, although that was nigh on impossible. Desperately needing to know that my body wasn't going to let me down, the fact that I was nearly thirty-seven years old was always

at the back of my mind. If only someone had a crystal ball and could have told me that everything would be OK. All these extra 'ifs'. How naive I'd been, thinking that pregnancy would be the end of the stress and anxiety. It was supposed to be a relaxing and happy time, but so far everything had proven to be way more intense than I'd ever imagined. Sometimes I did actually manage to adopt a 'que sera sera' attitude but, needless to say, that didn't last very long. I just found it too exhausting trying to subvert the natural thought process.

The bleeding had continued for a couple of days then to my surprise suddenly stopped – the nurses mentioned that I'd probably find that happened at some point. However, unfortunately it was short-lived as the bleeding returned on Thursday. Once again, my emotions took a battering and as soon as I let myself believe things were on track, I was thrown straight back in to despair and panic. I was slowly coming to understand that I couldn't take anything for granted whatsoever.

I found myself back at the hospital on Friday afternoon for another scan. I'd called the doctors' surgery in the morning, and after explaining that the bleeding had returned my GP called the Women's Centre to arrange for me to be seen again. Given I had a multiple pregnancy and was an older mother at the ripe old age of thirty-seven I was considered a priority, so there was no problem getting an appointment for the same day.

As I was called back into the scan room I tried to centre myself and steady my nerves. Those few days free of any worry once the initial bleeding stopped had been a joy, and I was so desperate to get that feeling back so I could really live the only pregnancy I was ever going to experience.

The sonographer had already reviewed my notes from the previous week and as I made myself comfortable she cheerfully said she'd try and see what was going on so she could reassure me that everything was going to be OK. She smiled as the cold jelly medium was squirted on my abdomen for the second time. "Here we go again," I thought. I couldn't look at the screen as it had been turned away from me, so I tried to study the sonographer's face as she clicked away with the mouse. After a few minutes of observation she gave me some tissue to wipe away the jelly, and began to explain what she'd found.

Smiling all the while, she told me not to panic as it didn't seem to be a serious issue, but she had seen a very small haematoma adjacent to the upper twin. My heart sank and off went my head again, thinking the worst. Amazingly I managed not to cry, and pulled it together enough to ask her some sensible questions. I wanted to know why there was a bleed, whether it was a common occurrence and when she expected it to stop. The answers to all three, unsurprisingly, were that she still didn't really have any. The only thing she could confirm was that it didn't look serious, and that sometimes there was a small bleed around the placenta, even on singleton pregnancies, but that often the blood is absorbed and the woman doesn't even know. Unfortunately for me, I wasn't one of them.

All the sonographer could do was assure me that both heartbeats were strong, and the measurements meant the due date was on track, signifying that both babies were growing well. That was some comfort at least, although I knew I'd be walking on eggshells until the bleeding stopped. In two weeks' time I'd be into the second trimester, and as I'd already researched miscarriage and birth rates, I knew that if I managed to get that far then, according to some of the pregnancy websites, the risk would drop significantly down to around three per cent. Although I wasn't daft enough to think that there was a magic date when everything would automatically be OK, I knew that getting to the second trimester was a milestone with regard to miscarriage. The psychological impact alone would be enough to ease some of the panic.

Once again I left the hospital not much the wiser about the 'why', although I now knew where the bleeding was coming from. "Hang on in there kids," I thought, "We'll make it. We're not coming this far for it to all end in tears."

Monday, 17ᵗʰ July 2006

After a weekend of surprisingly minimal panic and incredibly hot weather I had my first appointment with the midwife. It was also my first 'weigh-in' – 72kg, or approximately 11st 3lbs. I wasn't overly concerned with my weight – I had a very healthy diet, Pot Noodles aside, and ensured I didn't eat too much junk and sugar, so I knew that anything I did put on would all be baby related. Apparently, the average weight gain overall for twins was around forty-five pounds, or three and a quarter stones – now that was a scary figure!

The midwife also took my BP, which was an ideal 106/66. I told her that I still had some slight blood loss, but didn't have any pain, which she was very happy about as it meant that whatever was happening inside wasn't getting any worse.

We also discussed several tests that were usually done at this point – one was HIV and the other was something called the triple test, although I didn't need to have the HIV one as I'd had it done before starting the fertility treatment. The triple test is when the mother's blood is screened for levels of three different hormones that could indicate abnormality of some description, depending on the result. The midwife explained that there's a degree of inaccuracy with the triple test which is increased in multiple pregnancies, meaning that I could get a false positive, even though there could be no problems. To me this didn't even require any consideration – I didn't want to have a test that wasn't accurate to then risk further anxiety and worry on top of existing stress if it came back positive. I declined both the triple test and the HIV.

There was another test called a nuchal scan, which also assessed risk of chromosomal abnormality, including Down's syndrome. It was done by measuring the thickness of soft tissue at the nape of the foetus' neck by way of an ultrasound scan. The ideal time frame to do it was between eleven and just under fourteen weeks, and as I was about to cross over into the eleven week mark we needed to decide whether to have the test or not.

Depending on the outcome and given my age there was also the option of having an additional test called amniocentesis. This would involve taking a sample of fluid from around each amniotic sac via a needle through my abdomen, which would then be tested for any chromosomal disorders. Although commonly performed it was quite an invasive procedure and brought with it a risk of miscarriage of around 1:100[v], due to complications.

These were both very serious tests and needed our full consideration. We'd already discussed the amniocentesis to some extent, and given the long road we'd gone down to get to this point, I was adamant that I didn't want to do anything that would risk me having a miscarriage. The situation with the bleeding had reinforced that decision all the more for me. If it turned out there was a problem there would be nothing we could do about it anyway. As I'd be eleven weeks pregnant in three days' time, we decided to go ahead with the nuchal test but declined the amniocentesis, regardless of the outcome. We were booked in for the appointment ten days later – the twelve week mark exactly.

Thursday, 27th July 2006

Twelve weeks pregnant. I breathed a sigh of slight relief. I'd reached that crucial point and was considered to be in the second trimester – woohoo! I'd actually felt quite normal for the last ten days, even though I'd still had small bleeds on and off for the whole time. It had finally got to the point where, after so many instances and nothing happening as a result, I'd gone all cavalier about it and accepted that whatever was going to happen, would happen. There was no other option really, or I'd have sent myself completely doolally. I was happy that my brain had decided to kick in at last.

So, with another milestone complete we focused on the day's event – the nuchal scan. We decided that as it was such an important scan and we'd find out the results of our risk for abnormalities there and then, James should be with me when it was performed. I didn't want to be on my own if it turned out that the risk was suggested as being high, as I knew that would just set me off panicking again. Not that

I wouldn't do that with James being there, but at least I'd have another voice of reason and some comfort to hand.

Once at the hospital we sat and waited for ten minutes or so, then were called in to the scan room. The sonographer began by explaining that we'd actually be able to see proper outlines of the babies, although they'd only be around two inches long. Even though we'd seen the very early confirmation scan it was still very nerve-wracking to know that we'd finally be able to see that there really were two babies in there! Physically, it still wasn't apparent that I was actually pregnant as my belly hadn't changed at all. On the one hand I was quite pleased about that, but on the other I really wanted to have seen some obvious evidence by now, as it would have gone a long way to making it real.

However, there was absolutely no way I could have anticipated the feeling that came over me when I did finally see those baby-shaped images. I was completely speechless. At the click of a mouse the two 'its' became two real little potential people. At that moment, my world shifted once more and the reality and recognition of responsibility hit. I hadn't expected that, not at this point. The thought of it still being possible for something to go drastically wrong came flooding back, although this time it was accompanied by a steely resolution to carry my babies for as long as I possibly could.

In the haze of wonder I'd momentarily forgotten what we were there for, as the sonographer stopped clicking the mouse, turned to us and said that everything looked perfect. She waited a few moments for the data to be processed, then the printer whirred away and out came the risk report. It was broken down into two sections – the first one gave all the measurements of each twin, along with confirmation that various body parts and organs had been seen on the screen, and the second gave the estimated risk for Trisomy 21 (Down's syndrome), 18 (Edward's syndrome) and 13 (Patau syndrome). The sonographer took us through the report, where we saw that twin one was 57mm in length with a nuchal translucency of 1.4mm, all anatomy visible and appearing normal, and twin two was 51mm long with a nuchal translucency of 1.6mm, again all anatomy visible and appearing normal.

The estimated risk was based on a background risk factor dependent on maternal age, which was then adjusted based on the scan findings. My background risk for Trisomy 21 was 1:182, with an adjusted risk for twin one of 1:976, and twin two, 1:680. My background risk for Trisomy 13 + 18 was 1:319, with an adjusted risk for twin one of 1:2975, and twin two, 1:2221. The cut-off level for high risk was approximately 1:150, so given my results I was considered low risk. Another milestone checked off, another step forward, and another huge relief. Next stop – the gender scan.

Monday, 7th August 2006
Thirteen weeks, three days. We got through the last ten days or so with no huge drama but I wanted to check about a small problem that had arisen in the meantime so I'd requested an appointment with the midwife at the GP surgery. One day the previous week, directly after I'd woken up, I turned to swing myself out of bed when suddenly a sharp pain shot through the top of my legs and made me cry out in shock. What the hell was that? It felt a little bit like

I imagined fracturing a bone would feel. I got up and walked to the bathroom, but on every other step a milder version of the same pain went right through me again. I thought that it must be something to do with my body adjusting to the pregnancy, but I had no idea exactly what was causing it. For once I didn't panic – my gut feeling told me it wasn't related to the babies. It was difficult to pinpoint the actual source of the pain though, as it radiated in an arch through my legs and pelvis. It wasn't debilitating but I wanted to find out the reason why it was happening.

I sat in the nurses' office as the midwife took my BP – 108/60 – and listened to the babies' heartbeats, both of which sounded good. I tried to explain the pain and she immediately nodded her head in recognition. It was something called SPD (symphysis pubis dysfunction), or pelvic girdle pain. The sacroiliac joints at the back and the pubic symphysis at the front of the pelvis hold it steady during activity involving leg movement. However, pregnancy changes the musculoskeletal position and function, and with the increasing weight load and hormonal changes the ligaments soften, causing the joints to become more flexible. From my description of the pain, the midwife was sure it was the culprit.

She gave me a leaflet that explained how to manage it – common sense type of advice such as being careful when moving your legs, avoiding strenuous exercise etc. Basically a complete waste of paper. I thought I'd be referred for physiotherapy, but apparently not – I just had to put up with it. The fact that I was only thirteen weeks pregnant and would only get bigger and heavier didn't seem to be a consideration.

The midwife noted our discussion on my record sheet, and that was that. She then said that as I was having twins, it was an IVF pregnancy and I was an older mother, she was going to refer me to the care of a consultant at the hospital, as well as being seen by the midwife locally. It was the first time that someone had mentioned some kind of extra support given my circumstances, and being under a consultant meant that I'd have lots of appointments with an expert at an early stage. Whilst I really wanted to keep ultrasound scans to a minimum, the consultant would be able to feel the position and size of the babies and, using a doppler, would double-check the findings of the midwife. What it meant in practice was that I'd see someone at least every two weeks – once a month each for the midwife and consultant. It was a good job I worked part-time and was able to arrange afternoon appointments.

The midwife called the hospital there and then to assign me to a consultant and make my first appointment. With a direct line through to the department she got through straight away and after a couple of minutes it was all sorted. I'd been allocated consultant obstetrician, Mr Lawrence Impey, who specialised in high risk pregnancies, and I was scheduled to see him for the first time three weeks later, on 31st August 2006. I left the GP's surgery safe in the knowledge of being intensely monitored, which gave me the chance to try and chill out. Just a little bit, mind!

Wednesday, 16th August 2006
Fifteen weeks exactly. We moved house over the weekend although it didn't go entirely to plan unfortunately; it was raining really hard all day, and the removals firm had

underestimated how long it would take to load the van, so they were still bringing in boxes at the new house at 11 p.m. I managed to escape most of the stress of packing as I'd been relegated to observer, but in the end I got so bored that I drove over to the new house, switched on everything that required it, then ended up in Tesco buying oven chips so that we could feed the removals men. James was absolutely shattered by the end of the weekend too – all the boxes that had been labelled with a specific room had just been dumped anywhere, so he wasn't best pleased to say the least, and neither was I. It took us forever to find out where things were and sort them out, although luckily my parents had arranged to come over for a couple of days to help unpack.

I was also due for my first appointment with a new midwife at my new GP surgery in Abingdon. I'd been feeling a little bit achy over the last week so really just wanted a 'listen in' with the doppler to put my mind at rest. I felt like I was being a bit of a pain to be honest but the new midwife, Marie, was really friendly and warm, and we had an instant bond; she told me not to be so silly and that given the circumstances she'd be just as paranoid. She told me that I could call her to arrange for a listen in any time I was worried.

She managed to find the two little heartbeats really quickly and I was immediately reassured. Something else she did that I wasn't expecting though was measure my fundal height, taken from the top of the uterus to the top of the pubic bone. Standard thinking is that it should match the foetus' gestational age in weeks to within one to three centimetres, so at eighteen weeks for instance, it should measure fifteen to twenty-one centimetres. At fifteen weeks exactly I measured around nineteen weeks – slightly over but to be expected, given there were two babies in there. I found it really interesting to learn about the biology of it all, although sometimes I wondered whether ignorance was a better option.

Friday, 18ᵗʰ August 2006
Fifteen weeks, two days. We drove up to my parents' house in Nottinghamshire on Thursday. After the house move we wanted some time away from all the disruption, and although my mum and dad had helped us with the vast majority of sorting and putting things away and we were pretty straight, we felt like a break from everything.

I also realised it was about time I started thinking about maternity clothes. I really wanted to stay in my 'normal' versions for as long as possible, but I knew that at some point rather soon I'd probably just balloon up overnight, then have to go to work with several buttons open and my belly exposed as my shirts no longer fitted. It was quite exciting in the main, although as soon as I started looking for maternity anything I realised that actually the selection was really rather limited. It was hard enough looking for clothes when not pregnant, what with standard sizes all being completely different. Some of the high street clothes shops stocked maternity ranges but more often than not the garments were made of some nasty polyester mix. It was a form of punishment itself having to wear unfashionable trousers and such, but resembling a parachute was a one-way ticket to frumpydom.

Anyhow, my mum, dad, James and I all set off for a

223

'boutique' maternity-wear shop located in the Broadmarsh Shopping Centre in Nottingham. It was rather aptly called Swells I think, but as soon as I saw the store my heart sank. It was tiny. How on earth would I find anything in there? I sighed resignedly, but we decided to go in and browse anyway. I didn't really know what I was looking for – a couple of pairs of trousers and some tops sounded about right; I really didn't want to buy a lot of stuff to only wear it for a couple of months. It wasn't as if I'd need it again in the future.

My mum and I looked through some of the rails, picking up an assortment of items as we went, although I nearly cried when I saw the prices. £100 for one dress – seriously? Yes, it looked nice and all that, but the cost was ridiculous. It seemed I could look half decent whilst making myself completely penniless, or have a bit of spare cash but look like a sack of potatoes!

Several sighs later I was in the changing room trying on a couple of things. I came out to show my mum and James wearing an unbelievably baggy chiffon top with ties at the back. There was no way I'd need to wear that – it was huge. My mum and I started giggling as I shoved a cushion up the front to imitate my future belly. The assistant grinned at us, "Did you say it's twins?" she asked, "In that case, believe me, you will definitely need it." "No way," I thought. "That's just obscene – I won't get that big surely?"

I thought about it for a while then on persuasion of the sales assistant decided to buy it, along with a couple of plain coloured tops. Although I didn't need it then, my sensible head told me I should be prepared for the third trimester.

It would be nice to have something pretty to wear at that point anyway, especially as it would be Christmastime. If I didn't use it I could just sell it on eBay or something. I didn't, however, bother to get any trousers – I'd already bought a couple of adjustable pairs so I could manage with those for the time being. On the one hand I was quite happy that I could wear some of my normal clothes for a bit longer, on the other though I secretly wanted my bump to start being a bit more obvious. As it was it just looked as though I'd eaten all the pies!

Wednesday, 23rd August 2012

Sixteen weeks. Yet another midwife appointment, but nothing much to report. I measured twenty weeks, so a little bit larger than the average but still completely ordinary for twins. My blood pressure was an impressive 100/60, with the twins' heart rates at 158bpm for twin one, and 140bpm for twin two. Apparently each twin would be around four to five inches long, and they could probably hear our voices by now too. That meant they'd also be able to hear Eros Ramazzotti seeing as I played his music non-stop both in the car and at home. At least they'd be more likely to have my taste in tunes by the time they arrived, rather than all that progressive rubbish from the 1970s that James favoured!

Work was stress-free and I was eating normally, even though it was usually fish, fish and more fish. Sardines, mackerel, salmon – I couldn't get enough of all those omega oils. So, a fairly peaceful week in all; it looked as though things had finally settled down, and I'd taken to walking round with a permanent grin on my face.

Thursday, 31st August 2006

Seventeen weeks, one day. It was my first appointment with the consultant, Mr Impey. When I arrived at the hospital I had to give a urine sample, then get weighed. Aargh – did I really want to know? I stood on the scales then told the nurse what the figure was. This time I was 78.8kg, or 12st 5.7lb. Blimey; I'd put on just under a stone in one month! Oh well, you had to laugh really; there was nothing I could do about it. It was all baby weight, or at least that's what I told myself. I knew I hadn't let myself down on the eating front – none of that junk food rubbish and stuffing your face with cakes for me. The only thing I hadn't been doing was vigorous exercise, just plenty of walking. The nurses didn't appear to think my weight was unusual though, as they recorded the figure on my notes. I'd also seen a very sudden and noticeable difference in my belly size, to the extent where I could no longer wear my usual trousers and skirts. It was weird as it just seemed to happen over the past couple of days.

My appointment wasn't in the Women's Centre this time, but in the main outpatients department. After I'd registered and been to the weigh-in I was directed round to the ultrasound room as I had to have a scan to check the length of my cervix. I got the impression from the nurses that there was a 'panic point' of 25mm, and anything less than that was highlighted as a red flag and potential preterm delivery. Fortunately mine measured 32mm so it was nothing to worry about.

Next stop the waiting area where, after handing my notes to another nurse, I was called in to a consulting room. I'd done what I usually did and taken a book with me in case it was a long wait, and I'd just read a couple of pages when in breezed Mr Impey. It was the first time I'd met him and he was very friendly, and clearly knew his stuff. After he examined me and reviewed the results of my scan, he confirmed that I'd have to attend his clinic once per month until my due date. He said that it was standard procedure for a multiple pregnancy as it's classed as high risk, regardless of the age of the mother. I was quite pleased that they were keeping an eye on me; it suited my tendency towards being a control freak!

Before I left, Mr Impey also wanted to discuss the date of the next big milestone – the anomaly scan. It was usually performed at around twenty weeks and as well as taking a close look at the babies and my uterus, it was the opportunity to find out the gender of the babies. I'd been thinking about it for a long time actually. Some people weren't bothered about finding out and wanted a surprise but I was absolutely desperate to know, if only to stop me referring to them as Meringue and Sherbert, which I'd been doing ever since the first scan. I wanted to connect to them as individuals before they were born, and be able to picture them being boys, girls, or both.

I reminded myself that there were an awful lot of women who either couldn't have treatment, or had it and experienced failed attempts, and I realised that it didn't matter at all what gender they were. It was such a privilege to be having twins too; I still couldn't believe just how lucky we'd been. I couldn't stop my head from thinking about it though, just a little bit. Two girls? Yes, I could do that, no problem. Two boys? I could see that being rather more of a challenge! One of each? Wow, that would just be the most perfect outcome; too perfect to even hope for.

Thursday, 21st September 2006

Twenty weeks pregnant, and I'd been daydreaming on the way to our scan appointment. The past three weeks had been bliss – no bleeding, no worrying, no major incidents. Apart from ever increasing pain from the SPD I was doing really rather well. There was now no mistaking that I was expecting, but rather than having a very obvious small and neat bump, I seemed to be getting very round sideways as well as front ways. It was probably normal when carrying twins, but I saw it being a problem once I started getting bigger. Another few weeks and I wouldn't be able to get my car seatbelt on. Mind you, if I was that big my belly would reach the steering wheel and I wouldn't be able to drive anyway!

I did need to think about practicalities though so I did some research and found something called a bump belt. It was a pad that you sat on with two Velcro flaps that wrapped around the lower part of the belt ensuring it sat underneath your bump. So, that was one problem solved, although I knew I'd more than likely be unable to drive my car at some point. That was another thing – it only had two doors. Manageable with one baby, nigh on impossible with two. A double pram definitely didn't fit in the boot, especially not with all the other paraphernalia that accompanied it. We had to start thinking about a bigger car.

I was jolted out of my daydream by the car's brakes as we stopped to wait at the lights in Headington – we were nearly at the hospital. We turned the corner on to London Road then James turned right into Sandfield Road a bit further down to check if one of the on-street parking spaces was available. We were lucky and managed to find one straight away, giving us plenty of time to get to the hospital.

We nervously made our way up to the second floor of the Women's Centre and the ultrasound department. I handed in my notes and we sat in the waiting area along with several other couples. I expected a bit of a wait, and I wasn't disappointed. I flicked through some magazines and James read his newspapers so it wasn't too annoying. After a while we were called through by a smiling nurse. As I sat on the ultrasound bed I could feel my heart beating, and that nervous empty stomach feeling reappeared – not so much gentle butterflies as great big flapping crows!

The sonographer began by telling us what she'd be looking for in terms of measurements and anatomy for each twin. She smiled then asked us if we wanted to know what gender the babies were if she was able to see clearly on the scan. I nodded and said, "Absolutely, yes," and explained that for the time being they were either called Meringue and Sherbert or twin one and twin two; I couldn't wait to find out!

The scan commenced as various measurements of each twin were taken including ear to ear, head and abdominal circumference, thigh bone length, and a few others. The anatomical checklist was there to ensure that the organs were all seen as present and correct, after which the position of each placenta could be determined. Happily, both twins measured as expected, no abnormalities were detected, and there wasn't anything that couldn't be seen on the scan. Phew. Next came the really exciting bit.

The sonographer notified us that she was about to check for the sex of each baby. It was incredibly nerve racking; almost as much as being back at the first scan when were told it was twins. A short wait ensued when time just seemed to stop.

James was stood next to me when we heard the first confirmation, "So, twin one, situated on your left in a head-down position is a boy." We looked at each other and grinned, happy that we were having a son. The room went quiet again and I stared at the ceiling as I silently repeated to myself, "Please, let the other one be a girl." I looked at James in expectation whilst the sonographer viewed the second twin, then, after twenty seconds or so I heard her say, "And you'll be happy to know that twin two, on your right and currently in a breech position…is a girl."

Monday, 25th September 2006

Twenty weeks, four days. My jaw ached from all the smiling and I'm sure people thought I was a bit barmy. In a state of shock once more, the last few days had been just mad. Of course, as soon as we were outside the hospital I was straight on the phone to my mum to tell her the news; she was ecstatic all over again! I felt incredibly grateful to be having one of each, and I still couldn't believe it. Suddenly it was as if someone had flipped a switch and these two little blobs became real little people. Our last chance and we'd been so lucky that the treatment had worked, with the now added bonus of an instant balanced family. The gratitude I felt towards University College Hospital was beyond words.

Although I yearned to let everyone know I also sort of didn't want to. When I'd gone to work the morning after we found out, my colleague, Ali, kept badgering me to tell her – she was desperate to know what sex the babies were. But I'd decided I wasn't telling; the only people who knew were my mum and dad, Anna and her husband Chris, and James's parents. We'd told family that I was pregnant at around the week thirteen mark and they were all very excited to learn that we were having twins, but we wanted to keep this little surprise back until after the birth.

So, at just about twenty-one weeks pregnant, I felt really good but a little tired. I did notice that my pelvis was gradually getting worse though, and it took even less movement to send those shooting pains right through me. I had to remember to swing my legs round together whenever I did anything like get out of a car, a chair, or bed. It wasn't completely debilitating however, and luckily I was still able to go to work as normal.

Thursday, 28th September 2006

Twenty-one weeks. I was sitting at my desk at work, ploughing through a pile of letters, when I felt something strange going on inside. It was difficult to describe but I would intermittently get these sensations like tiny bubbles popping in my abdomen. It didn't dawn on me what it was at first, but then after an hour or so it just clicked, and I quietly said to Ali that I thought I could feel the babies. I explained the strange feelings and she nodded in agreement, confirming that was exactly what it would be. It felt incredibly weird and was completely unexpected. I hadn't given it any thought before and no-one had discussed it with me either. It was like having another little surprise.

Once I started to feel the twins' movements though another fear set in – I knew I'd constantly be monitoring when I felt anything and for how long, and whether they were moving too much or not enough. With two of them in there I imagined it would get a bit crowded later on too, and had to brace myself for any future blows to the ribs!

I managed to finish work a little earlier as I had an appointment to see the midwife. I'd called the surgery in the morning as I felt a bit lethargic, and I also wanted to hear the babies' heartbeats again.

After I'd done the usual urine sample the midwife tested it there and then, and I was slightly alarmed to see a result of +1 for proteinuria (presence of protein in the urine), one grade up from normal. Proteinuria detected after twenty weeks could be an indicator of pre-eclampsia which causes high blood pressure and oedema (swelling from fluid in the tissues), and often meant admittance to hospital. My blood pressure, however, was 110/68, which was in the standard range and although the likelihood of pre-eclampsia at this point was slim, the midwife still wanted the lab to do a test, just to make sure. It would only take a couple of days to get the result back, so it wasn't too long to wait. Surprisingly, although a little anxious I didn't panic – that good old gut feeling told me the test wouldn't show up anything to worry about.

Friday, 6th October 2006

Twenty-two weeks, one day. Wow, where did all that heaviness come from? It was like I'd woken up and found a couple of bowling balls in my lower abdomen. The pressure on my pelvis had become almost intolerable, but there was no way I wanted to take any painkillers. A paracetamol or two would have been alright, but the general advice was to take them for the shortest time possible, and I really didn't see the point of only having a temporary fix so I was stuck with the pain until after the birth. Using painkillers also meant it would be difficult to feel if I was overdoing things, so I thought it would be better just to get used to it and rest as much as possible.

I had another ultrasound scan and appointment with Mr Impey, so that meant time for another weigh-in. It had been around five weeks since the last one and I had no idea what to expect. I stood on the scales and watched the numbers on the digital screen, seeing them flicker up and down for a second or two then finally come to a stop on 83.9kg, or 13st 3lbs. Goodness, that seemed enormous; I still had four months to go.

With the humiliation of the weigh-in over, I was shown to a consulting room where Mr Impey's colleague checked my heart rate, which was 110/60, and listened for the babies' heartbeats and movements, which were recorded as heard. I then had a short wait until Mr Impey himself popped in and also checked the position of the babies. He asked me how I felt and whether I was managing the SPD, so I told him that whilst the pain was increasingly getting worse, I thought I could cope for the time being. He was happy with that and my progress, and asked me to speak to a nurse on the way out to arrange an appointment for another scan – my cervical length would have to be checked again a week and a half later.

As I walked back to my car I thought about the many checks and appointments at the hospital. Having twins at my age was an occupation in itself, and incredibly tiring too. I looked at my watch as I turned on the ignition – 3.15 p.m. I thought I'd stop off at Mothercare on the way home to see if they had something called a support belt in stock. Mr Impey had recommended it as I was starting to feel quite heavy; the weight would put enormous strain on my back by the end of the pregnancy and apparently it could help to alleviate any pressure. Anything that made me feel a bit lighter was definitely a bonus.

Monday, 16th October 2006

Twenty-three weeks, four days. Well the support belt turned out to be a complete waste of time. I tried using it on and off for ten days or so, but after an hour of constant wear it started to dig in to my stomach. It was very uncomfortable and made me feel really hot. I'd also ditched a couple of pairs of trousers that had stretchy over bump panels as I found them far too restrictive. In the end I had two skirts and one pair of trousers that I kept washing. They all had expandable panels and buttons on them and I just hoped they were big enough to last.

Anyway, it was the day of my second cervical length scan at the hospital's Fetal Medicine Unit (a management unit for high-risk pregnancies, including multiples), located on one of the top floors of the hospital. The nurse told me when I made the appointment that they had better equipment on that level, so I was sent up there instead of the standard ultrasound department.

As I sat gazing out of the window at the view of Oxford, I realised how busy the department actually was – it seemed to be a hive of activity. As well as me there were at least three other women waiting, plus several others in the small ward just off the main waiting area. Apparently the department dealt with a lot of pregnancies that were at risk of pre-term delivery, and as I sat there I wondered how on earth those women coped with such uncertainty. Little did I know at that point that I would soon become one of them.

Chapter 10

The End and the Beginning

After half an hour or so's wait I was called through to the scan room. The sonographer asked me to remove my lower clothing and make myself comfortable on the bed then she disappeared for a few minutes. I glanced around the room and noticed that all the equipment looked a lot newer than on the lower floors. Mr Impey had mentioned that they'd get a clearer image by performing the scan on these machines as they were much more advanced.

The sonographer returned and explained the procedure then did a standard doppler scan to check the twins' activity, which turned out to be perfectly fine. She then did the cervical scan using a vaginal probe – apparently, it's easier to see the cervix properly and get an accurate measurement.

I waited and watched the screen as she performed the scan, although she'd turned the monitor slightly away from me so I wasn't able to see very well. I tried to read her face as she clicked all the measurements with the mouse but all I saw was concentration. When she was finished five minutes later she smiled and asked me to get dressed whilst she went to get one of the doctors to go through the results with me.

My immediate thought was how strange that was – I'd always been given the results straight away on previous occasions, but it looked like she didn't want to do that this time. Maybe it was nothing but it didn't feel right, and I recognised the beginnings of a slight panic in my stomach. I breathed deeply and slowly and told myself I was just being daft – obviously that was just the procedure in this particular department.

I didn't have to wait long before a doctor appeared, sat on the side of the bed and began to talk me through the findings. She said that she didn't want me to worry but the length of my cervix measured 19.6mm which was very short, and given I was twenty-three weeks and four days pregnant I was officially considered as having threatened pre-term labour.

I didn't hear the rest of what she said as I was trying to concentrate on not being sick. My head began to pound and my emotions started to get the better of me once more. I couldn't take it in – I couldn't believe it was happening. I had my little boy and girl inside me and the thought of losing them now was unbearable. "Please, please, please let me be OK," I thought. I was strong up to a point, but this had gone way past that and the all too familiar tears began to fall.

The doctor saw how distressed I was and led me out to the small ward where she sat with me while I managed to gain some element of composure. I kept apologising as I was a bit embarrassed by my reaction, but she was very kind and told me not to be silly and that it was completely understandable, especially after everything we'd been through.

Trying to encourage me, she then said that it wasn't all bad news and I forced myself to listen as she explained about the other findings on the scan. Apparently there was something else they looked for when pre-term delivery was a possibility, and that was called funnelling. It's when the cervix begins to dilate and efface from the inside, meaning that the body is having trouble sustaining the pregnancy. The positive thing was that there was no evidence of funnelling on my scan at all, and as I didn't have any cramps or pain, the only thing they needed to do was check me again two weeks later.

I sighed heavily, trying to process everything, whilst the doctor continued to explain that there were things they could do to try and get me as far along as possible including complete bed-rest, hospitalisation or even drugs. There was also something called cerclage; they could place stitches in my cervix to hold it closed, although it was rarely performed after twenty-four weeks as there was an increased risk of membrane rupture, premature labour and infection. I was twenty-three weeks and four days – it was not an option for me. All I could do was wait and hope that I at least made it to the third trimester.

Thursday, 26th October 2006

Twenty-five weeks. The past ten days had gone by in somewhat of a blur. After I left the hospital that Monday I headed into work and after a chat with my managers we decided that given the circumstances it would be best if I was signed off sick for a few weeks, until I reached the date when I officially started maternity leave. I was so grateful for their understanding; they supported me in doing whatever it took to keep both babies well.

However, it turned out that not being at work any more and James being in London was maybe not such a wise decision after all. I was left alone all day, which gave me ample time to get myself into a right old state. It would probably have been a good idea to disconnect the internet completely, because most of the time I found myself searching online for information and statistics about pre-term birth and survival rates in twin pregnancies. The possibility of losing one or both of them didn't bear thinking about.

I knew, though, that I had to force myself to try and remain optimistic – I was adamant that they were staying put. I felt a sudden urge to personalise them both too, given the circumstances. They had their own little identities already, and although we hadn't decided on names for them yet I wanted to call them something other than Meringue and Sherbert, especially as we knew we were having one of each. After a short deliberation I came up with a choice of Percy and Ada, or Stanley and Mabel, so I plumped for the latter. I don't know why I picked those; I just thought they were really cute, and whilst we didn't want to call them that once they were born those names really did seem to suit their personalities. I'd experienced a lot more activity from them too just lately including some breath-taking kicks to my ribs, and their heaviness and fidgeting meant that the SPD started to be problematic. It took me ages just to walk to the bathroom some days.

Anyway, today was appointment day for my weigh-in and check-up with Mr Impey. It was the first one since that awful day a couple of weeks ago, and it was amazing how I'd managed to survive the previous ten or so days without having a complete mental breakdown.

Whilst researching survival rates I'd found out that the point of what was called viability i.e. able to survive outside the womb, albeit in NICU[vi], was twenty-four weeks, and at that point approximately forty-two per cent of babies survived. At twenty-five weeks that increased to around sixty-six per cent, and then at twenty-six weeks, seventy-eight per cent[vii].

Naturally, if I hadn't been the one who was pregnant and had to comfort someone else in the same situation I'd have said that a forty-two per cent chance at twenty-four weeks was really encouraging. However, when it's you it affects it's different; forty-two per cent still wasn't good enough – it wasn't even a 50/50 chance. Not only that, but when I first found out I was at risk I was only twenty-three weeks and four days, and the difference within that one week period was dramatic – twenty per cent. It was an awful situation to be in and I took to living day to day, not daring to hope much further than the next twenty-four hours. Each day that passed was a day they became stronger and stronger.

I did, however, manage to reach twenty-four and twenty-five weeks with no further problems. In my head I absolutely had to get to at least twenty-six weeks, when the rate shot up to seventy-eight per cent, although I knew I'd be unable to really relax properly until I reached the thirty week mark.

So, back to my appointment. I stepped on the scales and discovered that I was 85.7kg, or 13st 7lbs – an increase of 4lbs in three weeks. Good news in itself really, as it meant that if I was getting heavier the babies were getting healthier. My blood pressure was amazingly normal too – 100/60, in spite of all the stress. Both fetal heart rates and movements were heard and tracked, so all was good there.

The next thing to do was get through another cervical length scan. I'd told James that I was happy to go on my own, even though there was a risk that things could have got worse in the past few weeks. This time I was aware that it was a possibility and if it was bad news it wasn't going to come as a complete shock, so I thought I'd be able to handle it.

Fortunately, this time I didn't need to. The measurement was 20mm; a change of a tiny .4mm in an upwards direction, and still no funnelling. Although it was only small difference I was so relieved – another obstacle was over. I knew I had to be strong and focus on each day and week as they came, as I'd had to do in the first trimester when I experienced the bleeding. I had to accept that it was what it was, and the only thing I could do was stay in the moment as much as possible. I was absolutely determined to reach thirty weeks at the very least.

Wednesday, 1ˢᵗ November 2006

Twenty-five weeks, six days. The fun had just started in terms of getting zero sleep. If I turned on my left side I got a kick or three from Stanley, if I turned to my right I got one from Mabel. It wasn't comfortable on my side anyway as my belly was getting increasingly heavy. I couldn't lie on my back either as it's not advised for pregnant ladies – it could compress one of the blood vessels in the legs and subsequently make you feel lightheaded.

I'd ordered one of those long body pillows to try and help support me with the additional aim of easing the back pain, but it hadn't arrived yet so I had to manage with four or five normal pillows in the meantime. It was just so inconvenient having to sleep all propped up and it felt completely unnatural. At this rate, by the time the babies arrived I'd be so used to the sleep deprivation it'd be a complete doddle!

Thursday, 2nd November 2006

I felt a bit funny when I woke up this morning. At first I thought it was maybe to do with my restless night but I also really didn't fancy breakfast, although I forced myself to eat some plain oats. I didn't feel ill or anything, just strange, and I had a weird stretched and tight feeling in my upper abdomen. James had gone to London as usual and I didn't have anything scheduled for the day, so planned to drive into Oxford while I was still able to fit behind the wheel. I knew I'd be completely reliant on other people in a few weeks' time, which would obviously mean having to stay at home during the week. I supposed the bus was an option but they weren't very regular in the village, and I'd have been bound by timetables anyway; it all seemed like too much hassle.

I made myself a quick lunch – it should have been a sardines day (I ate them at least three times a week), but I just couldn't face it so ended up with a sandwich instead, then got in the car, switched Eros on the CD player and drove the short journey to the city. When I arrived I parked in the main Westgate car park – it was the most central and meant the least amount of walking and I was conscious that whilst I needed some exercise I also didn't need to overdo it, given I was still only twenty-six weeks and not yet in the 'safe zone'.

I spent a couple of hours in Borders, reading the magazines and drinking my usual chai tea latte. It wasn't too busy in the week and you could sit for hours if you wanted to – a group of women from what must have been a local knitting club often hogged all the comfy chairs though. I couldn't be bothered to do anything else afterwards so eventually I made my way back to the car. I got home around mid-afternoon, then parked myself on the sofa and read a book for a while.

As 5.30 p.m. approached I thought about making dinner, but as I still didn't feel quite right I just had vegetable soup. By 7.30 p.m. I started to feel a bit odd again so went upstairs to put my feet up for half an hour. The plan was to nap for a while until James got home, but something I couldn't put my finger on made me quite restless. I went back downstairs to make a cup of tea, and as I switched on the kettle I felt a sudden need to go to the bathroom. I rushed to the downstairs toilet just in time, and was alarmed that I obviously had an upset tummy. I didn't have stomach pain as such, but I was slightly concerned so I called the number for the community midwife in Wantage.

After explaining my symptoms she said that although she didn't think it was anything to worry about, given I was having twins and I'd felt some type of tightening earlier on, she thought it was probably a good idea to go to the hospital just to get checked. It wasn't urgent and it would be alright to wait until James got home so he could drive me to Oxford, but in the meantime she advised me to have a warm bath; the water might help me feel better. I did get a bit panicky but as I had to wait an hour or so for James anyway I decided to do as she suggested. There was a bath on the first floor in the family bathroom but I didn't use it often as I preferred the one in the ensuite on the top floor.

It was bigger and nicely decorated and had a more intimate atmosphere. I could submerge myself in the warm water, light a couple of candles and try to chill out for a while.

At around 9 p.m. James finally arrived home and after I'd explained what had happened we set off for the hospital. It was about 9.45 p.m. when we arrived and were registered on the obstetric outpatients ward. We were taken into a private room straight away and I explained my symptoms to the midwife. She said that she had to examine me first then monitor the twins' heartbeats for half an hour, so she took my pulse which was 88bpm, my temperature which was thirty-six degrees, and my blood pressure which was 113/78. She recorded that I had no oedema then began an internal exam to check whether the membranes were still intact.

I assumed the 'smear test' position and tried to relax, but as soon as the speculum was opened up inside me I felt this immense knife-like searing pain, at which point I screamed rather loudly and nearly ended up on the ceiling, completely shocking the midwife. Luckily she was able to do the exam regardless as I managed to remain in position through gritted teeth, despite the pain, and she saw that my cervix was definitely closed. We were all a bit confused as we couldn't work out why the exam had been so painful for me, but I assumed it was because of the SPD. She apologised about hurting me then confirmed that nothing was out of the ordinary, and that she hadn't felt any tightening at the time. Two sticky monitor pads were then attached to my abdomen and I was wired up to the CTG[viii] machine for half an hour.

I looked at James who'd gone his usual shade of pale

at the sound of my protests. He seemed agitated but as I settled down with my eyes closed and tried to nap for half an hour, which was pretty difficult in a room with fluorescent strip lighting, he opened his book and began to make notes about something or another. It was a good job he'd brought something to take his mind off things, although it would probably have been a good idea for me to have done the same.

After what felt like only ten minutes but must have been at least half an hour, the midwife returned to review the results of the CTG. The printout showed that both babies' baseline heart rates were normal, and there was no evidence of uterine contractions. The consensus was that I just had a mild bout of gastroenteritis, and I was allowed to go home. I'd already lost count of the amount of times I'd felt relieved that something had turned into a nothing, and I left the hospital feeling much happier that anything serious wasn't about to happen.

Thursday, 9th November 2006
Twenty-seven weeks. It was cervical scan day again – I weighed 87.6kg, or 13st 8lbs, and my blood pressure was 110/70. Mr Impey was really pleased – the scan revealed a length of 21mm. For the 'nth' time I began to relax ever so slightly.

Monday, 20th November 2006
I spotted him as soon as he walked out of the main entrance to the railway station in Oxford. My brother, Mark, had come over from Germany to visit me for the week and I was so pleased to see him. We didn't get to see each other

that often any more and it was really nice that he'd come over before the twins arrived – I hadn't told him yet but I had a plan to rope him into building the two baby changing stations we'd bought, as James hadn't had time yet what with working in London. Luckily for me he was very obliging and two days later the whole street probably heard us arguing about which way round the wheels went and whether there was a bolt missing or not; typical brother and sister!

After a few days of sightseeing and shopping in Oxford and our parents coming down to visit, the week went by rather too quickly, and before long Mark returned home. I thought about the coming days as I approached the thirty week milestone, and the fact that my parents would also be leaving the country as they were going on holiday for a few weeks. They'd be on the other side of the world, pretty much out of contact, and I began to feel a little bit lonely.

Tuesday, 28th November 2006

Twenty-nine weeks, five days. I headed back to the hospital again today as I had another appointment, this time with an anaesthetist. My midwife asked me last time I saw her whether I'd had any thoughts about pain management during the birth, and I'd said that I was a bit confused as to what to do for the best. Whilst I didn't think it would happen I didn't want to risk having a 'general' if the birth turned into an emergency for any reason. She suggested that I meet with the anaesthetist so we could go through the options and what they would mean.

I knew I had to get my birth plan written down too, and pain control was something that I really wanted to be clear on before the event. I knew I'd be upset if anything happened that meant a general anaesthetic and I subsequently missed the birth completely. It was something that had been on my mind for a while so it was useful to get the professional's point of view. One option I considered was having the epidural catheter in place for the delivery but not activated or topped up during labour unless I needed it. It would mean that if the delivery didn't seem to be straightforward then the doctors could start to give an anaesthetic and top it up if I needed assistance or an emergency Caesarean section.

The anaesthetist agreed that my plan would be a sensible one then we discussed whether I also wanted to use gas and air. I knew I'd need that as a bare minimum anyway – I wasn't that brave as to even attempt giving birth with no pain relief at all. One other thing I really did want was a water birth but it was inadvisable with twins unfortunately so I agreed with the doctors on that point and accepted that it wasn't to be.

I was much happier once I'd made the decision on pain relief, and it got me thinking about the rest of my birth plan. Ideally I wanted as calm and non-interventionist a birth as possible, painkillers aside, and my plan reflected this with requests for dimmed lighting, my own music and massage with aromatherapy oils. The midwives probably thought I was a right old diva, but apparently those kinds of things were all completely normal and quite common.

The only thing I was slightly concerned about was the delivery suite itself. I'd already been on the hospital's labour ward tour to familiarise myself with the environment; something that all pregnant ladies were advised to do.

It turned out that there were only a few rooms with windows – the others were in a central position between two corridors. I noted that these were quite stark, the ceilings were very low, and to me they were rather depressing. Although it was possible to request a window room there was no guarantee I'd get one, as it depended on how many births were happening at the time. My naïve visions of giving birth in a lovely room with a homely atmosphere were completely dashed, and I had to get used to the idea that realistically, I'd be allocated one of the central rooms. I consoled myself with the fact that at least there was a dimmer switch – things often looked better in low light, pregnant with twins lady included!

Thursday, 30th November 2006
Thirty weeks; and breathe.

Tuesday, 5th December 2006
Thirty weeks, five days. Due to increased SPD pain my midwife arranged to visit me at home for my appointment. I think the doctors took pity on me given my walk was starting to resemble that of a ninety-year-old and my feet wouldn't fit in my shoes any more because they were all swollen. I thought I'd avoided the whole puffy ankle syndrome but sadly it was not to be. I'd also taken to wearing that maternity top I'd made fun of back in the summertime; it didn't even cover my bump any more! I thought I'd have to go outside wrapped in a blanket soon as well – trying to do up a coat was getting to be a complete waste of time!

We chatted for a while then all the usual measurements were taken and the babies' heartbeats were listened to.

My BP was still fantastically normal at 112/70. I'd started to get some oedema in my hands though, and I tried to explain how painful the SPD had become; it took me ages to get out of bed as I struggled to turn my legs after resting all night. I'd also tried to use the support belt again but just couldn't get on with it and had to take it off after an hour or so. Sleep still evaded me too, in spite of the large pillow I'd ordered.

Apart from all that I was fine, although I did feel isolated somewhat. It took a lot for me to feel uncomfortable being on my own, but not being able to go out in the fresh air and have the freedom to go where I wanted was rather trying. All my midwife could offer was her understanding really, and whilst physiotherapy had eventually been prescribed, my reduced mobility meant I couldn't attend any sessions anyway. I didn't let it bother me too much though. To be honest I was just extremely grateful that I was still going at just under thirty-one weeks. Both twins sounded very healthy and, thank goodness, the short cervix problem had turned out not to be one after all.

Wednesday, 20th December 2006

Thirty-two weeks, six days. It was only a few days until Christmas and I so couldn't be bothered to put up a tree. The thought of faffing about with decorations and whatnot when I had to lump such a great weight around was completely unappealing. In the end I attached a few baubles to a large floor-standing twig-like object I'd bought from Habitat or somewhere. It actually looked quite pretty with a few white lights on it.

Given my temporary lack of enthusiasm and as I was so immobile, we decided to have a quiet Christmas at home instead of driving up to visit both sets of parents – the worry of anything happening whilst we were away and then having to go to a strange hospital wasn't worth the risk. My parents were due to come down for New Year's Eve anyway; that would be plenty of socialising for me.

Today was also the last time my midwife visited before Christmas; it was really nice having the same one every time as we got on well and 'clicked' in terms of personality. She completely understood all my fears and was very supportive. Unfortunately there was no guarantee she'd be there at the birth though – you were just allocated whoever happened to be working at the time. I thought that was such a shame, but the NHS wasn't set up for a more tailored level of support. I'd have quite happily paid extra for it, but that wasn't even an option.

After she'd checked my BP – 110/80 – she listened in to Stanley and Mabel then explained that she had to take a couple of swab samples from me to test for something called GBS, or Group B Strep. It's a bacteria that can be found in the digestive system, and often in the vagina[ix]. Normally it's harmless, but if passed to the baby during birth it could develop into a serious infection. Not all women are carriers of GBS, but if found it can be treated by administration of intravenous antibiotics during labour. It would take only a couple of weeks to find out if I was a carrier or not, but in the meantime it wasn't anything to worry about.

Thursday, 28th December 2006

Thirty-four weeks. Getting this far is an important milestone for a twin pregnancy, when everyone on the medical team gets to breathe a sigh of relief. If the babies arrived at this point they'd probably only need to spend a week or so in NICU and usually wouldn't have any long term health issues.

Looking back on the potential for problems earlier in my pregnancy I was so happy that I'd come this far, even though I could no longer get my shoes on and was considering a wheelchair to get from the car to Starbucks! Seriously, the weight on my pelvis and the SPD pain was almost intolerable, but I was determined to get to the next milestone of thirty-seven weeks, when a twin pregnancy is considered full-term.

Anyway, I had a growth scan at the hospital in the afternoon, the results of which showed that both twins were on target; Stanley on the mean, Mabel slightly above it. I wasn't given their estimated weights but I knew they couldn't possibly be small. They'd been very active an awful lot lately too and you could see limbs moving around all the time, and make out the shape of feet traversing my belly backwards and forwards. It was the weirdest thing I'd ever seen and very funny. In terms of positioning they were both cephalic, meaning head-down, and it was the best position to be in ready for delivery. If they didn't show up before, my induction date was planned for some time shortly after thirty-eight weeks.

As for my health, my BP was still really good at 100/65 and I weighed an incredible 93.6kg, or 14st 7lb, and wow, did I feel it. I was actually doing rather well, apart from swollen feet and the SPD pain; both temporary issues that would subside eventually. I supposed I was extremely lucky not to have any stretch marks either, although I'm not sure how I managed to get away with that as they were very common. It must have been a reward for having to put up with such an elastic abdomen that would take forever, if at all, to ping back again. Not that the gym was calling – I had no interest whatsoever in getting back to a size 'x' or anything resembling it; that would come in time. Probably by the year 2020!

Thursday, 11th January 2007

Thirty-six weeks. The hospital scales weighed me in at 96.7kg, or 15st 2lbs. Blimey – I didn't want to look any more, which was a good job really because I was already struggling to put socks on given the view had long been obliterated. Apart from that I felt well, but I was also completely fed up. New Year's Eve had come and gone and although we were all excited about seeing the babies in a few weeks' time, my distress at not even being able to walk without shuffling did worry everyone somewhat.

During my appointment I told Mr Impey how difficult I was finding it physically. He studied my notes and charts for a moment then said he thought it was about time the twins put in an appearance. He arranged for me to be admitted to the hospital on Wednesday, 24th January at 3.30 p.m., ready for induction the following day. That was just two weeks away.

Thursday, 18th January 2007

Thirty-seven weeks. I'd arrived at the last milestone of full-term for twins and I was ecstatic that I'd managed to get so far. Although there was no sign of anything labour wise, I had experienced some strange tightening sensations over the past week or so. Being first-time pregnant I found it really odd – my whole abdomen would suddenly get really hard and tight, then relax, then do it all over again. It also looked like my bump had changed shape, so I wondered if one or both of the babies had decided to shift position. I mentioned it to the midwife who said the tightening could just be strong Braxton Hicks, or it could just be one of the babies moving. Both babies sounded great and had perfectly normal heartbeats. It turned out that they were both still cephalic too which was fantastic, as it was the perfect position for a vaginal birth.

The past week had also got me thinking about the induction process and whilst not exactly anxious, I was a little apprehensive about not being in control and not knowing what would be going on. My midwife told me about the process itself, which did go some way towards easing my concerns, although I still had reservations. Apart from that the last week had been fairly uneventful. I'd ensured that whatever needed to be prepared had been, such as changing the car which we'd picked up just before Christmas, and I'd remembered to do small things like getting clothing and bedding sorted and in the cupboards. I'd been pretty organised in the main and there was now nothing left to do but wait.

Wednesday, 24th January 2007

Thirty-seven weeks, six days. Well, this was it – the beginning of the end of the beginning. My mum and dad drove down to accompany me to the hospital to get booked in as James had a meeting he couldn't rearrange. Nothing was due to happen until Thursday anyway, and I'd see him later at evening visiting.

I was in a happy, positive and excited mood when we parked the car in the afternoon and made our way to the hospital's maternity ward where I had to spend the night. I hadn't slept well the previous night, understandably, as all I could think about was the induction. I'd been mentally preparing myself for this moment, trying to still my mind and ignore any impending nervousness.

We slowly walked over to the entrance, where several women were stood outside wrapped in dressing gowns, cigarette in hand. Pushing aside my annoyance that they were allowed to do that at the only access to the maternity ward, I held my breath for a couple of seconds until we were safely inside the building.

The admissions office was on level two, so it wasn't too far to waddle. I walked up to the glass-fronted counter, gave my name to the lady on the desk and told her that Mr Impey had booked me in for a twins' induction the following day. We were immediately shown into a delivery room where a midwife took my blood pressure – a standard 110/76. She left us alone for a few moments before returning looking extremely sheepish.

She explained that my name wasn't written down in the delivery suite diary for an induction appointment. I looked at my mum with raised eyebrows. "What was she going to say next?" I wondered. Apparently, although Mr Impey had requested my induction, the communication between the consultant's office and the delivery suite hadn't been actioned. Additionally, there was a backlog on the labour ward and there'd been a virus in the neo-natal unit, so the hospital wasn't accepting anybody else.

Feeling extremely hot and getting stressed and agitated,

a wave of nausea came over me and I had to close my eyes to try and remain calm. This couldn't be happening. I'd psyched myself up for several days believing I'd be induced on Thursday and now the hospital told me that, due to an error on their part, they were unable to admit me. I was incredibly upset, and all the midwife could say was, "sorry". I sensed a general attitude of nonchalance; that really it wasn't important and what was the problem? I could just come back on Friday. It felt as though there was complete lack of empathy for my situation. I thought it was supposed to be a caring profession?

I sat for a moment as if stunned into inaction. I realised there was absolutely nothing I could do about it; I wasn't going to be admitted after all, and that was that. My mum was absolutely furious and made her feelings known in no uncertain terms. She grabbed my hospital bag and we slowly walked back outside where my dad was waiting with the car. I tried to reason with myself by saying that it didn't really matter, but however much I tried to listen to my rational head, the emotional one kept taking over. It sounded silly but I couldn't quite shake the feeling that it was an omen of some sort. A tiny seed of worry had been planted, and it wasn't going to go away; my confidence in the hospital had been severely dented.

Friday, 26th January 2007
Thirty-eight weeks, one day. Waking up at home on the Thursday morning in familiar surroundings gave me time to think about what had happened the previous day, and presented the opportunity to try to gain something positive from it. My parents hadn't been able to stay over

on Wednesday night as they'd had to get back for work the next day, and James had gone in to the office as usual, having got up at the ungodly hour of 5 a.m., so I was left to my own devices once more.

I tried to get the whole episode in perspective. I realised that the most positive aspect was that Stanley and Mabel had been given an extra few days 'tummy time' so to speak, and that was fantastic from a developmental point of view. Although as twins they were considered full-term at thirty-seven weeks, as long as there were no issues any extra time spent 'in-utero' was a bonus. The fact that the neo-natal unit had been subject to a virus had also been a concern, so the extra days we'd been dealt gave it time to run its course. I realised I would have been in a complete panic if I'd gone in that day, had the twins, and either of them had needed the help of the unit. The single remaining niggle in the back of my mind was that I'd now give birth over a weekend, and as hospitals didn't tend to have the same level of staffing and specialist availability at that time I was worried that it could mean a higher risk of problems.

So, after yet another restless night I attempted to get myself in the right frame of mind whilst finding it surreal that probably by Sunday I'd have two babies in my arms. James had taken the whole day off given Wednesday's saga and because my parents were unable to come over until Saturday. I wasn't sure why the hospital insisted on admitting me the day before – I'd have been much happier if I could have just gone in on the Saturday morning, even if it was at 7 a.m. or earlier. I really wasn't looking forward to staying the night in there.

I spent Friday morning just waiting for it to go by and

by 3 p.m. when we got in the car to drive to the hospital, I was quite fidgety. I was eventually admitted at 4 p.m. precisely, and was shown to a small room on the sixth floor of the Women's Centre. A midwife did my observations and checked heart rates – both twins sounded well. My BP was 100/60, I didn't have any contractions and membranes were still intact. By the time she'd finished it was just after 5 p.m. James stayed for a little while longer then left for home when my meal arrived. I felt unsettled, probably from anticipation of the unknown, and although the midwife said I should get some rest as soon as possible that proved to be much easier said than done. After reading for a while I closed my eyes and tried to sleep, but my mind raced and no amount of sheep counting seemed to make any difference whatsoever.

Saturday, 27th January 2007

Before explaining the events of the next twenty-four hours, I would like to say that in researching labour for multiples, and reading through and gaining information from my hospital notes that I wasn't privy to at the time, I discovered certain elements that, if I had known about them, may have prompted me to consider a completely different course of action, or at the very least ask questions. However, given my trust in the medical profession, and the fact that I truly believed they did know best, it did not, perhaps rather naïvely, occur to me to ask about any of the procedures and the reasoning behind decisions made in relation to my particular circumstance. After all, I didn't want to be considered a difficult patient who wanted to tell the medical staff how to do their jobs.

Whilst I don't doubt for one minute that all actions were honestly implemented and everyone wanted my labour to be a success, it still made me wonder, after subsequently reading through labour-related research myself, why other options were not explained or suggested.

Thirty-eight weeks, two days. I must have nodded off sometime during the early hours of the morning as I was woken up by a midwife knocking at the door. She told me that the plan was to take me down to the delivery suite some time during the morning, so I called James to tell him to get to the hospital as soon as possible. After taking a shower and brushing my teeth, I attempted to quieten my thoughts to try and achieve a relaxed and focused state of mind. By the time James arrived I was excited, but calm. The stress of the previous few days had gone and I was able to concentrate on the present. The thought of attempting a vaginal birth with twins was daunting, but I was determined to try and make it happen.

1148 hrs

I was finally taken down to the delivery suite. Nothing was out of the ordinary in terms of my or the twins' health – they were both in the cephalic position with good heart rates, and my BP was 110/80. I'd already been hooked up to the CTG earlier on to make sure both babies were happy, so there was nothing to worry about in that direction. I'd also confirmed to the midwife that I hadn't felt any contractions, so if my cervix was what they called 'unfavourable' after performing a vaginal examination, she would administer a prostaglandin gel.

The method of defining an unfavourable cervix is something called a Bishop Score. During the exam, various elements relating to the cervix are assessed and the scores are added together to give a total, which then indicates whether labour is likely to start spontaneously or not. I'd read that the lower the score, the greater the likelihood of an unsuccessful induction.

I'd been advised about the process of induction, such as the administration of prostaglandin gel etc., but I wasn't told about the risks or chances of success, nor had it been explained to me that my condition was not particularly favourable. If I'd been made aware of this prior to the induction I may have decided to wait a while longer to see if anything happened spontaneously, or at the very least to give more time for my cervix to ripen, especially given both babies sounded perfectly well at that point. Regardless, I was booked in for an induction, so as far as the hospital was concerned, that was what would happen.

1240 hrs

After getting settled in the room – a depressing one without windows unfortunately – the midwife had to do the first vaginal examination so she could work out my Bishop Score. Although I knew it had to be done and it wasn't going to be comfortable, just the thought that I might get the type of pain I had the last time made me anxious. I tried to relax and kept saying over and over in my head that this time it would probably be alright. It was just one of those things before, and it wouldn't necessarily happen again.

As soon as the midwife began the exam though I instantly experienced that same searing pain. It may seem overly dramatic, but it honestly felt as though my pelvis was about to snap. I shouted out for her to stop; that I couldn't bear it. She was understanding, if seeming a little frustrated, and she gave me the impression that she didn't really believe me when I tried to explain how excruciating it was. She did, however, suggest that I use Entonox (gas and air) whilst she quickly tried again, and the second time around I was able to breathe through the pain. Marvellous stuff!

As far as the Bishop Score went, the notes on my labour record said that it was six – on the borderline of what was considered favourable. The midwife immediately administered 2mg of prostaglandin gel then started to monitor both babies' heart rates. It was then a case of 'sit and wait'.

1431 hrs

It took slightly over an hour and a half until I began to feel something, at which point I recognised painless tightenings approximately four times in each ten minute period. The painless element would not, I knew, last for very long.

1450 hrs

Both babies' heart rates sounded good when the anaesthetist finally arrived to have a chat about the epidural, although the tightenings had started to become more uncomfortable. The plan was to break my waters at around 1830 hrs, and given the amount of pain I'd been in for the vaginal exam a couple of hours earlier, we agreed that the best thing to do would be to give me a combined spinal-epidural anaesthetic 'top-up' dose beforehand. It would allow them to proceed without me getting anxious and distressed. I'd then only have further doses of the anaesthetic if needed, once things started to get going.

I had absolutely no problem with that whatsoever. In fact the tightenings were starting to turn into cramp-like pains already and were definitely getting stronger. Any notions I'd had of giving birth with minimal pain relief and being all Mother Earth and natural slowly faded away, and whilst I was slightly sad about it I was also a realist – I knew I'd need all the help I could get if I intended to push two babies out. In the meantime, James was bored to tears!

1605 hrs

Right – enough of the pretend contractions. They were five in ten minutes now, and lasted around thirty seconds each time. On a scale of one to five with one being period-type cramps and five being very painful requiring analgesia I estimated that I was somewhere around a three. My waters hadn't been broken yet and I wasn't in established labour either. I hoped that things wouldn't get any worse before the anaesthetist turned up.

In the meantime my parents had arrived so the midwives now had my mum and dad to contend with, as well as Anna and Chris who'd also turned up at a similar time. It wasn't permitted to have too many people in the room at any one time though, so the plan was for them to take shifts whilst the others took refuge in the relatives' lounge where they could relax and have a tea or coffee. Everyone's anticipation created a really weird atmosphere – after all this time we were finally going to meet our twins. If the average labour was anything to go by that could be around 3 a.m. on Sunday morning.

1630 hrs

Nothing much had happened apart from the pain that had gradually got stronger. James swapped shifts with my mum and we chatted to try and take my mind off being uncomfortable. The midwife tried to insert a cannula into my left hand, but was unsuccessful. I had no idea why it was necessary, but assumed it was because I was having an epidural line sited, and also because I was 'high-risk'. If anything did go wrong it was the quickest way to get any required medication inside me.

I looked at the clock – two hours to go until my waters would be broken. If this pain got much worse before then I didn't know how I'd last that long.

1700 hrs

The midwife had disappeared for a while. She'd been in and out all afternoon; clearly the labour ward was very busy. I thought that with twins the recommendation was that a midwife was present at all times, but obviously that wasn't the case. I did, however, really need something to ease the pain – it had got much worse and I knew I'd be unable to remain calm for much longer. My mum wasn't impressed that the midwife had left us and wanted to go and look for her, but I told her not to bother and to just press the call button instead. After a minute or so a completely different midwife appeared and I explained to her that I really needed some sort of painkiller. She suggested that I used the gas and air until the anaesthetist turned up.

I picked up the mouthpiece and breathed in deeply. I knew what to expect as I'd used it earlier on during the vaginal exam. After a few breaths I began to feel all floaty and light-headed. The effect was fantastic, but unfortunately it took only a few seconds before I began to feel normal again. I didn't want to overuse it as I knew it had the potential to make you feel a bit nauseous. Saying that I was really reluctant to put it down, now I'd got used to how pleasant it was. With only half an hour to go until the anaesthetist was due anyway, I decided there was absolutely no point in me sitting there in pain when I could do something about it, so I carried on periodically for the next thirty minutes.

1725 hrs

Things had picked up a bit. My contractions were one in every two minutes lasting for around fifteen to thirty seconds, although they were still not considered to be of the established labour variety. The twins were being continuously monitored via straps across my abdomen, and whilst they sounded perfectly happy it was quite difficult to pick them both up at times – they were a right pair of fidgets.

1726 hrs

I heard a knock at the door followed by the appearance of the anaesthetist. Yay! It was time to get serious about the pain relief. It did feel like I was being a bit of a pain and the midwives could probably do with a bit of relief, so quite timely really.

1737 hrs

I sat sideways on the bed and tried to lean over whilst pushing my back outwards so I was in the correct position for the anaesthetist to place the needle. Given the size of my abdomen that was a huge challenge but I managed it and it was over fairly quickly. My back had been numbed before the epidural needle was inserted so I didn't feel a thing.

1745 hrs

The anaesthetist gave me an epidural test dose. Perfect.

1800 hrs

It was time for the second vaginal exam and breaking of waters. Eek. To say I was a little nervous would be accurate, although with the epidural top-up dose I knew I wouldn't feel anything for a while so it wasn't a panicky type of nerves. According to my labour notes, by this time my cervix was soft and stretchy, being ½ cm thick and 2+cm dilated (externally 3+, whatever that meant). I did think that 2cm wasn't much but then maybe that was normal for this point in time with an induced labour. Nobody mentioned it so I just assumed it was OK. I did get the feeling I was in for the long haul though.

1805 hrs

Apparently it had been easy to break my waters and the resulting liquor was clear, which I knew was a good thing. For the time being that was all the intervention that was required. I still hadn't felt any painful contractions due to the epidural dose, but it started to feel quite difficult lying in a full lateral position. How I'd have loved to walk round a bit but with jelly legs it was out of the question. I tried changing positions and managed to alter the pressure slightly by tilting myself with the help of some pillows.

1815 hrs

We did another birthing partner shift change and Anna came to sit with me for a while. Moving positions had worked – I was very comfortable and couldn't feel a thing. Both babies were still doing well with consistently good heart rates, I'd started to relax again and I felt really positive about the impending experience.

The midwife told me she'd attempt to attach an internal heart rate monitor to Stanley if she found it difficult to keep track of him on the standard version. Both babies had been fairly active and the external monitors had already been re-sited several times each. I wasn't too happy about the possibility of having a monitor clip attached to Stanley's head though. I was also concerned about infections, especially given the new midwife had a streaming cold – was it possible that a virus could be introduced during the procedure? I didn't ask that question of course as it didn't occur to me at the time, but later on it became a huge 'what if?'.

1930 hrs

Not much progress unfortunately. Contractions were the same although I still couldn't feel them due to the epidural top-up. As time passed I also became really hungry. The midwife said I could have a light snack, although I thought I'd need more than that if they expected me to push two babies out for goodness sake. It wasn't advisable to eat too much however, just in case of an emergency C-section.

The latest plan from the doctor was to wait for at least two hours after breaking my waters before deciding whether to give synthetic oxytocin, which forces the uterus to contract. Another thing I wasn't told at the time was that it has the potential to increase the strength, length, and frequency of contractions[x]. As far as I remember I wasn't even asked whether I wanted it or not. In fact nobody even asked the question of whether I wanted the induction or not, and all of these 'stages' certainly hadn't been explained in terms of advantages and disadvantages.

2000 hrs

The epidural started to wear off at around five minutes to eight and the contractions were on their way to being intolerable. I wasn't going to be a martyr; there's nothing superior about enduring childbirth without pain relief. Then again maybe I was just being a wimp? Other women did it all the time didn't they? Or maybe not when they'd been induced. I had no idea and I didn't really care. "Sod it," I thought, "I'm having the top-up."

2100 hrs

A midwife finally gave me the dose just after 2015 hrs, so I'd been pain-free for around thirty minutes when I was told I had to have another vaginal exam. It had been three hours since the previous one so I was rather surprised to be told that absolutely nothing had changed – I was still 3cm dilated.

The midwife decided it was time to attach that electrode to Stanley's head but it couldn't pick up his heart rate, so she reverted to the abdominal version instead. I was a bit annoyed to be honest. I don't remember if they'd actually asked me, or if I'd given consent. Certainly nobody explained whether or not there were any risks involved, and I didn't see the point if they could pick up his heart rate anyway by using the abdominal transducer.

I was also told that in view of little progress, I was going to be prescribed the synthetic oxytocin, Syntocinon. Like all methods of induction, it could make labour much more painful[xi], and has to be given gradually to avoid too many contractions happening too quickly. Feeling completely out of control I had no option but to just go with it. Meanwhile, James looked rather exasperated – being a spectator and not having any input whatsoever was probably challenging.

2215 hrs

The administration of Syntocinon had begun at 2140 hrs, along with another epidural top-up just after. I was getting uncomfortable just sitting on my backside constantly, so I tried to move positions. Having to remain upright in the bed I had to keep alternating between tilting to the left then the right, just to relieve the pressure.

The latest CTG indicated that both babies were fine with accelerations but no decelerations. Accelerations are short-term rises in heart rate indicating fetal well-being, and decelerations are slowing of the heart rate which, if of the late variety, could indicate a problem[xii]. The continuous monitoring of the babies was certainly very reassuring, although at times it was difficult to pick up both heartbeats as they were still a bit fidgety, and my changing positions didn't help either.

I asked the midwife if she could dim the lights so I could attempt to get some sleep. Although the Syntocinon was working it would still be a good few hours at least before anything significant was likely to happen, so I told my mum and dad and Anna and Chris that they should go home. They agreed on the proviso that James would call them straight away if anything developed. Knowing my mum she wouldn't sleep anyway but at least it was an opportunity to rest, away from the hospital environment.

Sunday, 28th January 2007
0200 hrs

Sleep still evaded me during the previous few hours. Although very tired I just wasn't able to drop off, plus I was absolutely freezing which obviously didn't help, so the midwife gave me a blanket to try and warm me up a bit.

I had epidural top-ups at 2330 hrs and again at 0055 hrs. Each time the medication started to wear off I waited to see how long I could go before asking for more. I thought that the pain would get to a point then just settle there but it just got stronger and stronger, and the thought of enduring it for who knew how many more hours was unimaginable. No way would I have coped without those top-ups.

In the meantime, I'd had another vaginal exam to establish progress. By 0110 hrs, although still only 3cm dilated, I was fully effaced and the electrode was finally attached to Stanley's head. Whilst slow it was still a change in the right direction and I hoped we wouldn't have to wait much longer. The Syntocinon had been given at regular intervals too, so although I couldn't properly feel them I assumed my contractions were also getting more regular.

0235 hrs

My BP dropped a little to 96/62. I felt nauseous and began to shiver uncontrollably. Fifteen minutes later, at 0250 hrs, the Syntocinon dose was increased as I started to experience incoordinate uterine contractions; they weren't happening in a downward wave pattern towards the cervix, rather they were unsynchronised. The condition was associated with frequent, more painful contractions, with the pain persisting even after the contraction had finished[xiii]. Thank goodness I'd had the epidural.

0340 hrs

The midwife discovered that the fetal scalp electrode had fallen off Stanley's head, so it was back to the abdominal transducer which began to pick up his heart rate straight away. It seemed there'd been no need for the invasive version in the first place. Mabel's heart rate was tracked with no problem and sounded good, and my BP had picked up slightly to 100/55. I went from feeling freezing to very warm and I was hot to touch, with a slight temperature of 37.3 degrees.

0420 hrs

Contractions became more coordinated – five in ten minutes. The plan was to do another vaginal exam at 5 a.m. to assess progress.

0500 hrs

Contractions were unbearable again – I needed another top-up. The midwife suggested she did the exam first but I insisted that she wasn't going anywhere near me until I'd had the drugs. I knew for a fact that it would be too painful and the gas and air wouldn't touch it. Why did she suggest doing that? Hadn't she read my notes?

0511 hrs

With the top-up complete, the midwife checked my BP. Oops. Back down to 97/49. I needed fluids. And I was very tired.

0520 hrs

The vaginal exam revealed I was 4cm dilated. That was 1cm in four hours. The midwife informed the doctors but they decided to wait for another two hours, at which point they planned to check again for progress.

0615 hrs

When I said I was tired an hour earlier, I really meant it. I started to get a little bit upset. The pain of the contractions returned as the last top-up started to wear off, so the midwife advised me to make use of the gas and air until the latest dose of epidural took effect. It didn't help much at all though and I felt myself getting stressed. I was worried and slightly frightened and became a bit tearful. The midwife and James tried to reassure me but it just felt as though no-one on the medical team really knew what was going on or what to do, and any faith in the process that I did have slowly eroded away. It felt like I was last on the list when I thought I'd be given more care seeing as it was twins. Not that I expected special treatment, but I'd been led to believe all the way through my pregnancy that I'd be much more closely monitored and taken care of during labour, and what did I find? Midwives changing shift like it was going out of fashion, and forever in and out of the damn room. After seventeen or so hours the seemingly never-ending situation and the thought of something happening to one or both of our babies was all-encompassing, and from then on the panic really set in.

0640 hrs

I was given some paracetamol as I had a slight fever. Shallow decelerations had also been picked up, although I wasn't informed at the time and I don't know which of the babies it was.

0729 hrs

The midwife had gone AWOL again but as soon as she appeared back in the room I barked at her that I needed another top-up. I felt sick too so was also given an anti-emetic. Unsettled and starting to lose it, I didn't know what to do, which was a bit daft because I wasn't in a position to be able to actually *do* anything. Feeling completely out of control I looked at James who looked rather alarmed; I'd never seen him look so anxious. He'd had to sit and watch what was going on all night and I could tell he was angry and deeply frustrated.

0750 hrs

My mum and dad arrived to be greeted by me in a state of frenzy, having to use the gas and air to dull the most excruciating unspeakable pain I could ever have the misfortune to experience. That's the only way I can explain it because it was completely unexplainable. The top-up I was given at 0730 hrs hadn't been effective at all so apart from the gas and air I was coasting on zero pain relief. My mum was aghast to see me so distraught and kept asking why someone didn't just do something? Oh, and another new midwife took over.

0805 hrs

I'd had two top-ups in the space of half an hour. My BP had been consistently low for a while so IV fluids had been increased and it emerged that my uterus had been hyperstimulated with the Syntocinon, so that was reduced again. Not only was the epidural not working but over stimulation meant that the pain was so much worse than normal labour pains. I tried to concentrate on anything at all but regardless of the effort I put into it, I was just unable to find a place in my head where I could block it out, or at least manage it.

All this time not one of the midwives could understand why the epidural wasn't working, and nobody thought to check. It wasn't me, I wasn't going completely mad and I knew I had more of a threshold for pain. I was convinced that it shouldn't be this way but nobody on the medical team seemed to be listening. A doctor had at least been called to review the situation but they were all busy doing C-sections so I had to wait. Trying desperately to focus I felt any strength I had left quickly dissipate.

0840 hrs

With the epidural still not working I wouldn't let go of the gas and air and the mouthpiece was permanently glued to my face. As soon as the effects from the last breath had worn off the pain hit me straight back again. The room started to spin and it felt like I was stuck in one long never-ending contraction.

The doctor had already been in to see me and suggested that they attach the fetal scalp electrode to Stanley one more time. I also had to be examined again to see if I'd progressed or not. Initially I was so distressed that I just said no, but I knew they really did have to do it so had no choice but to agree. The problem was that I anticipated the pain from the exam as well as the contractions, so it took all my remaining strength to get through it.

Unfortunately, nothing had changed. In fact my notes said that I was only 3cm dilated when the check prior to it had been 4cm, and that my cervix was ½ cm thick when they'd previously said fully effaced! The doctor could feel that my uterus felt tense when it was supposed to be at rest, and Stanley had increased swelling on his head. The fact that both of the babies' heart rates were considered normal and reassuring was probably the only thing that kept me going. Against all my hopes and wishes for the birth of my children, I realised that there was absolutely no way I could carry on, regardless of the fact that I wasn't progressing anyway. There was no option – I sadly conceded to a C-section.

0910 hrs

It was very difficult for both my mum and James to see me in so much pain and distress. The anaesthetist had given me another top-up, but still it hadn't kicked in. I really, really couldn't cope for much longer. It was incredibly busy in the labour suite and as long as the babies' heart rates were fine I wasn't considered a priority, so I had to wait for a theatre to become available.

Feeling slightly delirious and with tears streaming down my face I kept asking James where the doctor was. I became more hysterical by the minute and felt nauseous and disoriented from all the gas and air. Finally the doctor arrived to tell me that a theatre was being prepared and to talk me through the consent form. I had absolutely no interest in going through anything, and I could barely talk properly anyway. I took the gas and air attachment out of my mouth, nodded my consent then scribbled my signature on the form and stuck the mouthpiece straight back in again. I closed my swollen, tear-stained eyes and just wished for the whole experience to be over.

The doctor disappeared out of the door and immediately the whole room went into overdrive. A porter rushed in with a bed to transfer me just up the corridor to theatre and everyone rushed around with a sense of purpose. I couldn't believe the sudden difference in focus.

As the gas and air was taken out of my hand and I lay down on the transfer bed, it was the first time I breathed in some proper air for quite a while and I felt my stomach turn. The porter and nurses wheeled me out of the room and as soon as they did, that was it; I had to be sick. Quite a lot sick. Deprived of the gas and air, I also became acutely aware of the contractions once more. The doctor told me that all I had to do was get through the next ten minutes or so and they'd be able to re-site the epidural and give me a lower body regional anaesthetic so I'd be pain-free. A midwife or anaesthetist assistant was with me the whole time, trying to take my mind off it whilst we waited. I felt like a complete failure.

0935 hrs

Theatre was a whirl of activity, and the amount of doctors, nurses and specialists was astounding – there must have been at least eight or nine people in the room. It seemed as though once you'd been defined as an emergency or they'd made the decision to operate, everyone became incredibly efficient. The difference was startling.

The anaesthetist checked the site of my previous epidural given it had seemingly not worked for several hours. And no wonder; it had fallen out and the tip was only just sitting in the space. I'd had no pain relief since around 7 a.m. that morning, and nobody had thought to check why I kept saying that it wasn't working. Unbelievable! I tried to get my head around the fact that I'd had both an induction and synthetic oxytocin, both of which were known to cause much stronger and more painful contractions than normal labour, plus been hyperstimulated which created unsynchronised contractions, causing yet more pain. How I hadn't passed out I just didn't know.

The anaesthetist finally re-sited the line and I was told that I would slowly begin to 'not feel' the lower half of my body. As I was infused with bupivacaine and fentanyl I slowly felt myself become more relaxed and less stressed. Gradually the local anaesthetic began to work.

In the meantime the midwife helped James get prepped and he suddenly appeared by my side – without his glasses and wearing a silly hat and gown as well as some equally daft-looking shoes. Ha! As I'd been in so much pain the least he could do was look ridiculous!

I asked him if my mum was coping, and was relieved to hear that she was taking it in her stride. Once I'd been wheeled off to theatre she'd calmed down a bit and had disappeared off to wait in the relatives' room along with my dad, Anna and Chris. In spite of the incredible pain and complete trauma of the past day or so I began to feel less anxious.

1006 hrs

After I'd been cleaned and draped the surgeon checked my reaction to make sure I definitely couldn't feel anything, then made the first incision. I was very, very nervous. It was as if time stood still whilst we waited to hear our babies' very first cries. The doctors talked to me constantly and let me know beforehand that whilst I wouldn't feel any pain I would probably feel some sort of tugging when they lifted each baby out.

My notes stated that Stanley was what's called asynclitic, which is where the baby's head tilts towards one shoulder. He'd been wedged in my pelvis and, being a twin, there'd been no room for him to change position. Nobody had any idea how long he could have been like that, but if it was for a while the Syntocinon would definitely not have helped – the resulting stronger contractions would have added more unwanted pressure. I didn't know if it had been the reason for my slow progress or whether it had nothing to do with it, but it was very upsetting just the same.

As the doctor pulled all 6lb 15ozs of Stanley out at 1010 hrs there were a few brief moments of silence before we heard his first very loud cries then, whilst he was being cleaned up the surgeon retrieved Mabel. She was born one minute later at 1011 hrs, weighing an equally impressive 6lb 11ozs, in good condition and screaming her hellos to the world! We were handed both our babies and, unable to contain myself, I was overcome by such indescribable raw emotion, more powerful than anything I'd ever known. All the past years of everything I'd experienced on the way to this moment came straight back. I was completely unprepared for the shock and intensity and could hardly see through the ensuing tears that flowed. Finally, I was able to hold our twins.

1100 hrs

Once sewn back together I was transferred to the observation ward along with Stanley and Mabel. The look on my mum's face when she finally saw the twins was priceless; she was overjoyed. I looked like I'd been dragged through a hedge backwards though, with huge dark circles under my eyes and a fixed look of utter exhaustion on my face. The remnants of the drugs were still in my system, along with some additional ones that were helping to alleviate any pain from the C-section.

I tried to breastfeed both babies straight away and it sort of worked in a fashion. For some reason Stanley didn't seem to be too bothered and just wanted to sleep. We all put it down to the trauma of the birth and having been stuck in my pelvis. He had this funny little kink in one of his ears and I wondered whether it might straighten out as he got older, bless him. Mabel was as quiet as a mouse too, and after she'd fed for a little while she snuggled her way up and under my left arm, right in to my armpit, where she remained for absolutely ages. It was like she just wanted to get back inside and go to sleep again. It seemed that neither of them were quite ready to be born when we rudely forced them out and into the world.

1530 hrs

Towards mid-afternoon Stanley appeared to be a little fussy and he started to make some strange little grunting sounds. His temperature was also down somewhat so the nurse placed a portable heater over his cot to try and warm him up. It worked, and by 1645 hrs he'd settled down. My parents and James went home not long after and

I attempted to get some rest in between trying to feed both babies. Left alone with my thoughts I assumed I wouldn't be able to sleep, but I was that shockingly drained that I didn't have any problem dropping off at all. The only thing that woke me was the return of the surgery pain and my subsequent request for painkillers.

Monday, 29th January 2007
0600 hrs

I awoke after a fairly uneventful night. Mabel was doing really well, but Stanley was still making those grunting noises and was quite mucousy. The midwife had being doing observations on him throughout the night and he'd had the heater kept on, which wasn't usual. I felt uneasy and a small concern raised itself in my head when I was told that the paediatrician had been called to take a look at him.

0700 hrs

I was completely alone when they told me; neither my parents nor James were due to arrive until a bit later. The nurse popped her head round the curtain to check if I was awake and, seeing that I was, sat down on the edge of the bed. Her face looked quite serious and I knew she was about to tell me that something was wrong. I just stared at her with wide eyes, feeling my heart starting to beat faster and trying to swallow despite the lump in my throat. Paralysed with fear, I didn't know what to do, I didn't know what to think and I felt instantly sick when I heard her say, "Try not to worry Tru, but the paediatrician is going to refer Stanley to the special care baby unit; we think he has pneumonia and he needs a lumbar puncture."

Epilogue

Saturday, 3rd February 2007

I stood at my hospital room window on the fifth floor, staring out at the dark February sky. Dressed for the cold weather and with my bag packed and ready to go I felt a conflicting set of emotions whirling round inside me. There'd been a deep joy on the one hand and a spiralling fog on the other, and I was left feeling absolutely spent.

I'd been in the hospital for just over a week and I couldn't wait to leave it behind me. The pure happiness of holding my twins after the trauma of labour had turned into the uncertainty of the Neonatal Intensive Care Unit. I'd been dealt another round of complete emotional turmoil and I had, unsurprisingly, been diagnosed with PTSD (post-traumatic stress disorder).

I heard the lock turn on the bathroom door and my mum reappeared. She looked at me and asked, "Are you ready?"

I nodded my head and said, "Yes, I'm ready."

I turned around holding Mabel, who was quietly sleeping in my arms. James took my bag and opened the door for us. I looked down at Mabel then glanced back up again seeing the look on my mum's face. Stanley was in her arms gazing up at her and my heart leapt as

I witnessed the magic of my twin stars.

My mum looked at me as I smiled and softly said, "Let's go home."

Endnotes

i   Toni Weschler (2003). *Taking Charge of Your Fertility*. Revised edition. United States: Vermilion

ii   http://www.hfea.gov.uk/fertility-treatment-options-reproductive-immunology.html

iii   Agnew, C; Klein, A H; Gannon, J A. *Twins!: Pregnancy, Birth and the First Year of Life*. HarperCollins Publishers Inc., 2006

iv   BUPA   http://www.bupa.co.uk/individuals/health-information/directory/m/miscarriage

v   BUPA http://www.bupa.co.uk/individuals/health-information/directory/a/amniocentesis

vi   NICU Neonatal Intensive Care Unit

vii   EPICure http://www.epicure.ac.uk/overview/survival

viii   Cardiotocography – the monitoring of the fetal heart rate and uterine contractions

ix   Group B Strep – www.gbss.org.uk

x   NHS local induction and acceleration (augmentation) www.nhslocal.nhs.uk/story/features/induction-and-acceleration-augmentation

xi   Nottingham University Hospitals inducton of Labour (IOL) leaflet (pdf) www.nuh.nhs.uk/media/912009/0110v20210_induction_of_labour.pdf

xii   Interpretation of the Electonic Fetal Heart Rate During Labour; Amir Sweha, M.D.; Trevor W. Hacker, M.D.; Mercy Healthcare

Sacramento, Sacramento, California; Jim Nuovo, M.D., University of California Davis, School of Medicine, Davis, California. *Am Fam Physician*. 1999 May 1; 59 (9): 2847-2500. www.aafp.org/afp/1999/0501/p2487.html

[xiii] *Midwifery: Preparation for Practice*; Sally Pairman; Sally K. Tracy; Anna Thorogood; Jan Pincombe. Pg824. Churchill Livingstone

Lightning Source UK Ltd.
Milton Keynes UK
UKOW04f1219260913

217984UK00002B/4/P